Testimonials for 11 Points of Healthy Ageless Living

I first became aware of Mike Greer over thirty years ago at a convention in Austin. One of the programs was presented by a sports trainer, who was trained in a new way to measure body fat. He called for several volunteers from the audience to measure. When he got to Mike, he couldn't believe it—Mike's body fat was less than ten percent which is in the range of professional athletes.

Since that time, I have worked in the same industry as Mike and have become a good friend. When I try to describe him to people, I use words like "unique", "unbelievable", even "maniac". At over seventy years of age, he shows very little of the telltale signs of aging, due in part to the fact that he is an ultra-athlete, who trains every day. Couple that with a healthy diet and positive attitude, and you've got a zest for life that is truly refreshing.

But you can't describe him without realizing the balance that he has in life. He juggles several business interests, family, book writing, a web blog, and of course his triathlon training—and he does a pretty fine job at all of them. Through his vision, he showed the world of triathlon that Lubbock is a great venue to showcase the sport.

When he spoke to me about his new venture, I told him I wanted to help in any way I could. So, I'm writing this to tell you that Mike Greer can change your life— for the better.

Steve Moffett
General Manager,
Lubbock Electric Co.

I met Mike Greer a number of years ago while serving on the board of a Lubbock area non-profit organization. Mike's experience in leading organizations through times of change and uncertainty was critical to the organization's survival. He provided insightful advice, steady leadership, and was willing to make hard decisions at a time when there were plenty of difficult decisions to be made. Mike lives the leadership principles that he has espoused for twenty plus years—hard work, physical and mental fitness, creatively thinking about solutions, and listening to others.

While Mike is best known by many as a triathlete, those who know him recognize his true gift is his ability to coach, teach, and mentor. Amazingly, he has coached, taught, and mentored everyone from a fourteen-year-old from the wrong side of the tracks to national class athletes to political and business leaders. In sum, Mike understands that everyone is important and worthy of learning what it takes to achieve peak performance.

Personally, I have applied many of Mike's leadership principles in community service, while serving in Iraq and Afghanistan, and as a senior military leader. I am honored to call Mike a friend and appreciate deeply what he has shared with me about leadership.

Darrell Guthrie
Brigadier General
US Army
Attorney

My name is Lisa Ramirez. You and I met a couple of years ago while I was presenting a short half-day presentation for the City of Lubbock on multi-cultural issues. I have since moved to the Washington, DC area so I haven't been in Lubbock very often since then. I don't expect you to remember me—but at that time you gave me a copy of your book and I promised to read it. Well, I have! I started it and then I couldn't put it down. I am sure that you may have made the connection to such books as The Secret by Rhonda Byrne and some writings by Deepak Chopra. I was sharing what I had learned from your book with a person at work and she led me to a book entitled The Cosmic Power Within You by Joseph Murphy—written in 1968!!!

I say all this to say, that I am in complete agreement with your book and wondered if you had considered what an absolute gift your book has been to others. I am currently writing my dissertation on spirituality and its role in the lives and work of educational leaders and your book has really motivated and inspired me to stick with the study.

Well, I'll keep this message brief as I am not sure you will ever receive it—if not, well, I still feel better for having said thank you. If you do receive it, then I look forward to hearing from you.

Sincerely,
Lisa Ramirez

TRANSITION YOUR AGING TO MATCH YOUR MINDSET!

11 POINTS *of* HEALTHY AGELESS LIVING

MIKE GREER PhD

SEVEN TIME IRONMAN FINISHER & LIFE COACH

COVER DESIGN BY WANDA BAILEY

TRANSITION YOUR AGING TO MATCH YOUR MINDSET!

11
POINTS *of*
HEALTHY AGELESS
LIVING

MIKE GREER PhD

SEVEN TIME IRONMAN FINISHER & LIFE COACH

COVER DESIGN BY WANDA BAILEY

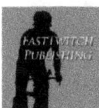

FastTwitch Publishing

Published by FastTwitch Publishing

Published in the United States of America

ISBN:978-0-692-90175-5

Acknowledgments

A special thank-you is extended to all those who helped me in making this book possible: to Larry Crosby, for working with me on getting it done and especially for giving me a deadline. Thanks also to Terry for proofing and Marti for typing. *It got done!*

Contents

Contents

Foreword

Healthy Aging
Unhealthy Aging
Not Aging at all

Of the three, I'll certainly take healthy aging. If there is anyone to guide you on this journey, it's certainly Mike Greer (or just Greer as most of us call him.) I became aware of Greer through the sport of triathlon almost fifteen years ago. At race after race, I saw a guy who was fitter, faster, and more successful than I was and seemed to defy the laws of aging. As the years ticked on, Greer and I had more opportunities to interact, and I realized that he was much more than simply an accomplished athlete. Greer epitomizes the term "self-made man."

While recently sitting at dinner, something became abundantly clear to me—Greer gets his drive and purpose from remaining *vital*. His almost singular focus is living for the contribution to his family, his friends, his clients, his community, essentially everyone he interacts with.

This is a powerful lesson for all of us as we continue the aging continuum—*stay vital*. What was the province of thirty- and forty-somethings a few decades ago is now open to sixty- and seventy-somethings. Sure, the body may not have the same kick as it used to, but the mind can remain razor sharp well into (and beyond) what we used to affectionately call "old age." Keep contributing in any and every way you can because not only does it benefit you, it benefits society.

As I prepare to exit the back end of the definition of "middle age" in a few more years, I no longer think about or fear death. What I do fear is going to the grave with too much value left inside me. I've accrued a lot of knowledge and experience in my lifetime, and I'm driven to share it wherever it will do some good.

So, let's then age in as healthy a manner as we can. We can keep the body strong, the mind sharp, and the contribution flowing. Let's redefine what "old age" means and what's expected of those who reside in it. I'll do my part if you do yours. I already know that Greer is doing his.

What do you say…are you ready to march bravely into your future?

Me too, let's go. Peace.

Michael Giudicis

Introduction

Since I have blogs that have been written starting in 2005 about every topic one could imagine, some good and some bad, some useful and some not, I have decided that after I have finished one of my eleven points, I will insert certain blogs from 2005 that may have application for the subject. How they fit into the subject matter may not be extremely obvious, but it will give the reader the opportunity to read it and decide for themselves if it has any application.

My point in writing my *Eleven Points of Healthy Ageless Living* is to offer some form of hope for enjoying the aging process and make it a more enjoyable time of life. Plus, people younger than I am are always asking me, "What is your secret?" I am providing the secret answers, which really are not secrets, in my own way and hope they ring a bell somewhere. The healthy aging myth is not a myth and has substance; it just must be articulated in such a manner that everyone "gets" it! It has been said that aging can bring on many undesirable things in life such as depression, anxiety, lack of meaning in life, and just simply wondering, "Where do I fit in?" Recently, a friend sent me the Senility Prayer: "God, grant me the senility to forget the people I never liked anyway, the good fortune to run into the ones I do, and the eyesight to tell the difference." So, let's get on with it!

What a privilege it is to be asked to write the *Eleven Points of Healthy Ageless Living*. During my lifetime, I have been asked many times, "What is your secret to looking younger than you are and being much more active than most people of your age group?" When I was in my early forties, most people would guess me to be in my late twenties.

When I was younger, I never thought much about it, and I sure never dreamed that the question of my age and health would be something that I would write about. But as I have aged, I have found that aging is one of the most popular subjects on the planet.

As I list my eleven points, I like to point out that I have always emphasized that I feel like my life has been really blessed in so many ways. Real wealth is determined by your health. While I have tried to practice those things that help me to be healthy in my daily life, I am no different than the average human being in that I have had to practice discipline in my life to provide my *Eleven Points of Healthy Ageless Living*!

I encourage everyone around me to establish their own eleven points, since not all would agree with my eleven and would feel better with their own. Recently, in a presentation of my Eleven Points, I asked for comments from my audience concerning their eleven points, and I found that there were some who wanted to add more to the list or replace some. So, this is what I encouraged each to do. As you read my eleven points, please be thinking about your own and write them down!

The good news about anything that is associated with a numerical beginning is that there always must be a number one. So, the number one on the eleven points of aging will be one that I know will stand out and deserve the number one rating. But I must add that all the eleven points are really just as important as the others.

If I made out a drawing of a pie and put the eleven numbers in each slice, I would make all the slices the same dimension. The truth of the matter is when I wrote out the first rendition of the "secrets" to healthy ageless living, I did this on a paper napkin in a small diner in Albany, Georgia. This was not some kind of luncheon honoring me and asking me to speak. This was a lunch with a representative of the City of Albany Chamber of Commerce trying to sell me on locating my cotton industry branch in Albany.

So, after the burger and well into the chocolate sundae, this person asked me what my secret of staying healthy, active, and useful is. My age at the time was around fifty-eight, and I sure didn't consider myself that old, but I answered her question by writing it down on the paper napkin. I thought this was kind of cool since I know of many businesses that have experienced a birth on a paper napkin, Southwest Airlines to name one.

The other truth of the matter is that I only came up with seven points and that stayed the norm for a while. Then one day, I was asked by a local Rotary Club to come and talk to them about my secrets to looking younger than I am, and certainly staying more active than many of my peers. As I looked at the original seven, I could see a need to add some new secrets to the list, and it came to ten. Then after I made my presentation to the local Rotary Club deep in the oil-producing Permian Basin of Odessa, Texas, I offered a Q&A time after the conclusion.

What I found was complete enthusiasm for the subject matter, but also some suggestions on other important points of life that left me with eleven points when I concluded the Q&A. To this day, I have given the eleven points to numerous groups, aging from fourteen to eighty-five, and the interest and response has been tremendous.

It is a fact that most of our population is very interested and obsessed with this thing called aging! One of my favorite books that I have within my personal library is that of Dr. Andrew Weil. His book *Healthy Aging* is one of the most complete and optimistic books available on the subject. While he is trained as a medical doctor, he also brings to the table a very open-minded approach relative to alternative or holistic approaches to healthy aging. He offers a complete lifelong guide to our physical and spiritual well-being. Such subjects as antiaging medicine, why we age, the denial of aging, and the value of aging are covered completely, and in a manner that the layman can understand.

He concludes this book with his twelve-point program for healthy aging. As I compare my eleven to his twelve, I see some points in mine that are not in his, and his twelve are presented in more of a general way, whereas my eleven are more specific and apply to my definitions and applications within my lifestyle.

I am a firm believer that all humans are created differently from the original DNA of their parents, so even though we may have some similar thoughts and physical appearances as others, we are still unique. The verification for that statement is simply exemplified by the fact that all human fingerprints are unique. Also, at this time, I would like to challenge my readers to look at their parents as if they are looking into a mirror and realize that what you see is a strong blueprint of how your healthy aging can be boosted by studying the DNA of your parents.

As you look at this, please take note of all the positives and negatives of your parents and realize that this can give you some plus and minus indicators of your life to come. Plus, you can observe the aging consequences of both parents. I declare right now that while we cannot change our DNA, we can positively affect it for the better through positive lifestyle actions, such as exercise, nutrition, psychological exercise, and a positive attitude for all good things in life.

As we view this mirror, we do not need to get down and depressed since I know for a fact that we can alter the DNA parental outcome by lifestyle changes or actions. While my father had colon cancer, prostate cancer, open-heart surgery, cataracts, etc., and my mother suffered from high blood pressure, alcoholism, and died of a massive stroke at sixty-five, rather than feel myself destined to these dreaded health problems, I faced them straight on with lifestyle habits that I know would combat these health issues in my life.

My challenge to my readers is to look at healthy aging as a major event in life with lots of positives. What I have found to be the greatest challenge in my aging process is the ability to transition my lifestyle both mentally and physically to fit the changing trends in our society. Since the computer age has fast forwarded our society in all things that we do, it is more of a challenge to make these transitions and realizing that what many call the "good ole days" are gone forever, and to enjoy life, we must harness the negative thoughts of progression and grow with the present.

My goal in life has always been to remain flexible and roll with the tide concerning change and advancements in our society. Sure, I can sit around and talk about the days of no cell phones, no social media, no computers, etc., but the fact of the matter is if I, or anyone else, want to continue to have some kind of involvement in the current times, there must be a willingness to learn new things or meet new people who can get some of the things done that some of us are not gifted or trained in.

I remember when I was in the manufacturing business in the early 1990s, and to build my equipment for the cotton industry, I had to hire class A welders to be able to produce high quality equipment. Since I had no clue on how to weld steel or any other metal, it was imperative that I hire welders to get the job done.

So again, I had to be flexible in my thought processes and not get discouraged because I couldn't weld. In my current multisport production business, I have seen the marketing practices change almost ninety percent in that the social media is used now rather than print, and the use of cell phones and computers is a must. That being the case, I have hired three social media people to do my marketing and use online companies to run special marketing campaigns to generate immediate business.

Another reason that I like to share my eleven points is because I can talk about them, and it may provide good suggestions for living a healthy lifestyle. What I have found is that aging is a big topic for most people, and as we age in an "ageless" manner it generates curiosity.

A few years ago, I was on a bicycle ride in the canyons with a group of much younger triathletes. As we climbed the hills many times and then did speed work, a young man came up beside me and asked my age. At the time I was sixty-eight, and I was kicking his royal butt, which prompted his question in the first place. I then asked him his age, and he said thirty-eight, so this gave me an opening to suggest that he should start planning his aging right *now* and not put it off.

When you wait until you're in your sixties, it might be too late at that point. On the other hand, I never discourage anyone from getting on the fitness wagon no matter their age. After my father had his heart attack and open-heart surgery in the middle 1960s, he *then* decided he needed a better diet and exercise plan. He was able to live a much better lifestyle the last fifteen years of his life. If he had changed his ways when he was in his early forties or fifties, he would probably have lived many years more.

With that in mind, I am going to move into my *Eleven Points of Healthy Ageless Living* and present a narrative of what they are and how they have influenced my life. I would also like to offer a voice of flexibility for these eleven points since I know as we age, these can change with the times as I've mentioned above. But I feel they can offer a strong baseline or foundation for all that we experience in our lives. What I get excited about when I see them is that they have application for everyone, and no one is excluded. They may vary somewhat from person to person, but for the most part, they apply to all our physical and mental needs and desires.

In addition to my eleven points' explanations, I would also add other caveats to this by adding some of my blogs that pertain in some way to the point.

In 2005, I started writing on my blog sites, www.fasttwitchmind.blogspot.com and maturefitness. blogspot.com, and after reviewing them, I have found that many have some form of application to my eleven points, so they will be added at the conclusion of each point. The years for the blogs will be given, and each person who reads this can tie in the significance of the blog to the point. In some cases, it might be subtle; others, right to the point.

My intention would be to create some thought processes into each point with actual everyday stuff, since all the blogs were written to make a point, even if humor or fiction was applied to make my point. The *Mature Fitness* blog was written with only fitness stuff, so it is limited on the number of blogs since its inception.

Here goes.

CHAPTER 1

Mythical Age

The trick is growing up without growing old.

—Casey Stengel

Mythical Age: If you didn't know your birth date and for sure didn't know your age, how old would you think you are? The first time I heard this remark was from my dad, and at the time he was seventy-five and he asked me this question. He told me he came up with that idea when many people he met during the day would ask him his age, and when he told them, they would comment he looked much younger.

So, based on this thought process, I have come up with what I call the mythical age that we sometimes think about. This could be a time in your life when everything was either going very well, or maybe it came after a challenge in life, or maybe when you had finished your formal education and was entering your career. My mythical age is twenty-eight, and really, the only reason I say that is because when I ask myself this question, that is the age that pops into my mind. One of the things I have done is a life chart from my birth date, which I do know, to the present, looking at it every seven years. In most cases, if we look at our lives this way, we will see many major things that have happened about every seven years.

As I consider the age of twenty-eight as a really good time in my life, I would guess if I could have stopped the aging completely, it would have been that age. This would also be another way to determine this age. My reason for having this in the magic eleven is because I have good feelings and believe that not only was this a very positive time in my life, everything around me was in the same shape.

"Lowe's Success" 4.19.2011

If you didn't know how old you are, how old would you think you are? Good question and while I know most everyone know their birth dates, I think this question can be used to analyze why aging becomes such a big deal. It seems that aging or growing old is the big topic of many conversations. Just this past week I was invited to speak at the Lowe's Wellness Center in my old home town of Littlefield, Texas, about my *11 Points of Ageless Living*.

Lowe's happens to be owned by my longtime friend Roger Lowe, Sr. and he has done an outstanding job of building this company and employing some really good people. Even though the company has grown into a multi-million-dollar company he has kept his corporate office in Littlefield and continues to grow with increased sales and expansion. Not only that he does it with a great philosophy of honesty in his dealings and state of the art business principles. It is so good to see this type of business, and to think Roger and I have been friends since the fifth grade and even played football together through Junior High, High School and College.

We were both raised by business parents and received great training from them with entrepreneurial spirit taught to us from the very beginning. They always taught us to be ourselves and never waver from that. I can say regardless of the financial success Roger has earned he has never wavered in being his true self. What a guy and what an organization he and his employees have built. Now, the answer to my question! If I didn't know my birth day, I would guess my age at twenty-eight. Now you got it, thanks for asking!!

Notes:

CHAPTER 2

Nutrition

The only way to keep your health is to eat what you don't want, drink what you don't like, and do what you'd rather not.

—Mark Twain

Nutrition: When I first started giving the eleven-point presentation, I would call number two Diet, and then one day, during the Q&A part, a nice senior lady stood up and said, "I don't think number two should be labeled diet, and it would be better served if you called it nutrition." Since I always listen to my audience, I decided to change it.

While nutritional practices started in the Garden of Eden (remember the apple?) it seems like it only really became a solid subject. There was a time when people would simply eat whatever was put in front of them without any concern to what it might do to their bodies. Can you imagine what a meal was like with the cavemen? People tended to "live to eat" instead of "eat to live," and there was no concern as to what true nutrition was. Which also makes me wonder why the bad foods were put on earth to start with! But I guess, philosophically, making life easy with no challenges would not be the Lord's way. Some basic words help define my balance of nutrition in that I use the forty percent complex carbohydrates, thirty percent protein, and thirty percent fat, and depending on the status of one's weight generally, 2,000 calories a day is adequate. Before any type of nutritional changes are made in daily food consumption, I would suggest that a trained, certified nutritionist be consulted. Now this can vary a little bit, but for the most part will take care of your nutrition needs.

It should also be noted that athletes may require more than the norm, but again this should be determined by a trained nutritionist. Different sports require more or less of a good thing to provide fuel for the body to make it through certain challenges. In preparation for an Ironman Triathlon, I decided I needed a refreshing evaluation of my daily nutrition to include my training and race day needs. Since this involved a 2.4-mile open water swim, a one-hundred-twelve-mile bike ride, and then a 26.2-mile run, I felt I should look at my nutrition a little closer than I have in the past.

In my younger years of competing, I was able to overcome the challenge of the distances, weather, and the unknown that happens when you are racing for up to seventeen hours (the cutoff). So, my nutritionist had me submit a seven-day record of everything I ate or drank in the quantities that I consumed them. From that, she was able to determine what I was good and bad on! Turned out my protein intake (very important for maintaining strength during events) was good, but I was a little short on my omega-3 and needed more vegetables. That was for my everyday nutrition. And then for training and race day, I would need lots of rehydration and complex carbohydrates for energy. At the end of this training and event, I would venture back to my normal nutrition with the addition of the veggies, etc.

Bottom line here is that nutrition has always been a big part of my life, but I still strive for the eat to live theory and always watch my weight. As we age, we must be aware of what we are eating—from quantity to quality—there is simply no excuse for not taking care of ourselves in this way. There is so much information out there now; it is just a matter of paying attention, researching, and implementing good nutritional habits. I recall in my college football and track-playing days, I would sometimes vary my weight by twenty-five to thirty pounds. depending on the sport I was competing in. The first year at the University of Houston, I reported for football training camp at one-hundred seventy-five pounds. and within two weeks, the humidity of the Houston area lowered my weight to one-hundred-fifty. That was my weight for the entire football season.

Turns out it was perfect for track, which I competed in during the spring. Then I reported back in the fall and was able to maintain a one-hundred-eighty pounds. playing weight. While my football weight was needed to play that game, it sure wasn't needed for the rest of my life. So, I have worked hard to keep a good nutritional plan and helped my health by eating what is good for me. It is just as easy to eat healthy as it is to eat unhealthily.

Of course, the other point here is to eliminate any of the bad habits in our lives such as tobacco, too much alcohol, drugs (prescription and illegal), fat, calories, and anything that that does not blend well with your body. Too much of anything, good or bad, can be detrimental to our health. I believe very strongly that while we have some great medical resources, *we* must take control of our lives and be responsible, doing everything we can to maintain a healthy lifestyle. We can help the medical profession by exercising some of our own due diligence and then putting into practice what can help our good health.

In previous generations, the usual practice was to wait until something is wrong with our bodies, before going to the medical profession to fix it. Kind of like the local auto mechanic who fixes your auto when it goes bad. Instead of that philosophy, we should take charge of our lives and health while doing everything we can to stay healthy. To me, the proof is in the pudding, when I hear of real-life success stories of people, I know taking charge of their life and health.

A close friend of mine had let his unhealthy lifestyle cause an episode of congestive heart failure while he was exercising. While he was saved with emergency procedures, he still had many unhealthy obstacles standing in the way for a healthy lifestyle. While the medical profession was able to save him during a medical emergency, it was going to have to be up to him to change his lifestyle to guarantee a continued active life. Well he did do this, and now he is exercising (walking, playing handball, lifting weights, etc.) and eating well, with no alcohol being consumed in his diet. He has lost sixty-six pounds and is feeling very good, and at the age of sixty-one, he is on his way to a healthy life of enjoying his work and family.

Jim Patterson, former Odessa Permian MOJO football player, I am really proud of you and congratulate you for taking charge of your life. You are making healthy ageless living a reality!

In *Healthy Aging*, Dr. Weil devotes a complete chapter to the anti-inflammatory diet; even though he likes to emphasize that rather than call it a diet, he prefers to call it a healthy nutrition plan that should become part of our lifestyle. This plan offers the ideas on how to select and prepare healthy foods. He states that inflammation is a common root of many chronic diseases and wrote about oxidative stress as a pro-inflammatory process. To get a bird's-eye view of the way of providing your body with great nutrition for all reasons, check out the web site, www. healthyaging.com. If you buy the book, you can check out Appendix A for complete details.

Invariably, the question of supplements comes up during this part of my presentation to various groups, and it is a good one. While there are thousands of supplements out there that are all supposed to be the best and most effective for your good health, I have found that it is very important to exercise as much due diligence as possible when it comes to taking supplements.

My first remark is to emphasize a good balanced diet with the 40-30-30 formula as mentioned above; however, I do confess that for the past sixteen years, I have been taking a supplement I feel is very good for my health and may even give me a chance for a longer healthy life. There are all kinds of descriptions out there like organic, natural, real food, whole food, etc. The most complete supplement company I have found is a twenty-year-old company by the name of Mannatech. Certified personal fitness trainer and eating psychology coach Ashly Torian endorses the Mannatech product line and says that eating organically-grown whole foods is the best way to avoid harmful pesticides, fungicides, and herbicides.

But despite our best efforts to eat healthy foods, we need to supplement our diets with essential vitamins and minerals.

Supplements made from natural, plant sourced vitamins, minerals, and glyconutrients are best, and that is why the Mannatech health, wellness, weight and fitness products are so good for our health. Regardless of what brand a person uses, I suggest that a person look for all the healthy features that are offered by companies like Mannatech. It is easy to research and study with just a simple "google it" exercise!

When I read the following blog article, I published a few years ago concerning one of the Select Milk Producers dairies that I was doing marketing work for, I am reminded of my teenage nutrition. While my nutrition then was completely controlled and provided by my mother, the one thing I insisted on was having a full quart of whole milk during the meal. I have always said the sum total value of anything in life results by evidence of the proof in the pudding idea! Well the proof in the pudding concerning my good health and strength in the bones is now personified by my consumption of this great product.

Whenever I might get injuries relative to the given sport I was competing in, I always experienced faster-than-normal recovery. It has been especially evident as I have aged. Within the past three years, I have had injuries in bicycle and motorcycle crashes, and in both, my doctors have said that I healed with the speed of a young adult. I then tell them about my whole milk experience when I was younger, and they just shake their head and comment it must have made the difference.

That is another reason I feel so compelled to share my *Eleven Points of Healthy Ageless Living*, since I know the points have worked for me and possibly will help someone else. But as I have also mentioned, it is imperative that life should be planned for aging, since that is the most effective way to insure a healthy senior lifestyle.

"Dairy Farmers, My New Heroes" 8.16.2011

When I was ten years old my grandmother taught me how to milk a cow. That day stands out in my mind very well and I remember her putting on her bonnet that farm women wore then and commenced to show me how to milk. She had two cows, so I had one and she had one. She showed me how to sit on the stool, place the bucket and then how to get that milk out. Little did I know that over sixty years later I would be associated with the dairy farming industry and how interesting it really is. The dairy farmer is truly remarkable since they must provide so much synergism in the process of getting their cows to produce good quality milk. They really partner with these amazing animals. The good news for me is that I am able to learn from the real professionals of this industry and every time I visit a Select Milk dairy, I learn something new.

This past week I was given another tour of the Legacy Farms just North of Ransom Canyon, owned by the Bouma Family. These folks represent a long history in the dairy business dating back to the early 1900's in the Netherlands, so they really know their stuff. The tour was conducted by Brad the Elder, and son Brandon and what I saw was extreme professionalism and pride in their dairy operation. It wasn't just about milking the cows and selling the milk, but it included extreme care in the way the "bovines" were cared for, with tender loving care.

As Brandon said, "when you check into a hotel you want clean sheets, clean towels, and a clean room each night you are there. Well that is the way we treat our cows, we take care of them and then they take care of us by producing quality milk." So, their pens are kept immaculate and their diet is watched over with a careful eye. Reminded me of a Marriott! Since the cows are milked three times a day, they must eat a lot, rest a lot, pee a lot, and poop a lot. Then they yield that healthy milk with tons of calcium, magnesium, potassium and vitamin D. What a package of healthy ingredients.

As we made that one last swing through the pen area where 13,000 head of prime Holstein cows were doing their thing, I swear it looked like they were winking at Brad and Brandon as we drove by. These guys were very happy, and you could feel that they enjoyed their work. Thanks Legacy Farms for producing many heathy milk products, Athletes Honey Milk being one of them, for the world to enjoy!

"Bad Boys of Food" 10.23.2010

While it has been some time since I have posted on the Mature Fitness blog, I thought it was about time to get something going. It is not like fitness has taken a stand still in my life or in my priorities. I have just been traveling too much and not really having the time to do two blogs and do them right. It has always been my goal to offer some new thoughts and insights to the idea of "mature fitness" but other things have prevented me from doing that.

On the other hand, during my travels I have become even more aware of the obesity that exists in our country, especially when I see people who cannot sit in one seat on the airplane and the overabundance of food consumed at the numerous all you can eat places that are available. Funny thing is the all you can eat places have some good healthy food but not in the volume they are available in. There simply is no reason for a person to eat the huge amounts of food that are available, so that is the main problem.

No discipline in food choices or amount, no exercise, and eating too much of the wrong things will lead to obesity. Simple as that, the principle of too much fat in and not enough activity to burn it leaves the fat in the body and then it is hard to burn off and keep off. The smart approach is to watch everything that goes into the body and use some restraint. In the case of the mature food consumer it is even more important to watch volume and type of food eaten since metabolisms do slow down with aging. Choosing the right foods and especially the volume of food is critical to good health and will help prevent obesity. Recently I saw a list of the six worst for you fast food items and was amazed at the calories and fat grams in the following bad guys of the fast food category, here they are:

1.   Arby's Roast Turkey & Swiss—looks innocent but it has seven-hundred twenty-five calories, and eight grams of saturated fat. Not the worst on the menu but did make the list.

2. Subway Foot Long Sweet Onion, Chicken Teriyaki—yea I know, Subway is well known for the huge weight loss of that young man that is used in the commercials. But remember, this is a commercial and he is being paid to eat right and lose weight. So, take all of this with a grain of salt. He did lose all that weight, but he was also paid to do this and was furnished with the most weight conscious food. This foot long of food has eight hundred calories and nine grams of fat.

3. Cinnabon Caramel Pecan Bon—1,100 calories, fifty-six grams of fat, and is the real bad boy of this list. Even cutting it in half would not be a good thing. I suggest that you get three of your friends, order one of these and cut it in four slices.

4. McDonald's Filet O Fish—this dude kind of drags you in with the thought of fish being a good thing; however, it is fried, put on white bread bun, then smeared with tartar sauce for a grand total of three-hundred-eighty calories, and eighteen grams of fat. Along with this you are tempted with a bag of French fries and then the calories really begin to climb. If you took this same Filet O Fish without the bun, no tartar sauce, and broiled it you would cut at least two-hundred calories.

5. Burger King Tendercrisp (means fried) Chicken Sandwich—eight-hundred calories, forty-six grams of fat.

6. Taco Bell Volcano Nachos—the name says it all and it really is a volcano for your stomach and bad to the bone. It has 1,000 calories, sixty-two grams of fat, but does also offer you sixteen grams of fiber which helps you get rid of this mess from your system.

An Honorable Mention to the All-Star list of bad foods is the Bread Bowl Pasta from Dominos—1,460 calories, and fifty-six grams of fat. Wonder why it didn't replace the little innocent Filet O Fish with only three-hundred-eighty calories.

Other funny note is that I have noticed that when people who are obese or need to lose weight, they always drink diet Coke. This is not good for the Coke folks since they don't work, which they don't. My solution to this obesity problem is very simple, cut back to half of what you are eating, add twenty percent more exercise and then make it a life style thing.

"Vitamin D Importance, Aging Can Be Fun" 11.6.2011

Vitamin D: My sources say the hottest new healer now is Vitamin D, yep that same ole vitamin that is called the "sunshine" vitamin. Lack of this sunshine vitamin is linked to cancer, heart disease and diabetes—and at least one third of the population does not get enough. So, how do we go about getting enough of this little jewel?

It is hard to get enough D through food, since there just isn't much out there except in mushrooms that are rich in D. Fatty fish such as salmon can provide some Vitamin D but when it comes down to it, ol' sunshine is the real source. Okay now you say, well what about skin cancer dangers?

Well just like anything you can get a good safe dose with five to ten minutes of midday (10:00 a.m. to 3 p.m.) sun on your arms and legs.

This will provide you about 3,000 IUs of D to a light-skinned Caucasian. Getting that amount two to three times a week is enough for most, but those with a big deficiency may need it daily. Adults up to age seventy should get six-hundred IUs of vitamin D a day, and those over seventy should get eight-hundred IUs a day. Vitamin D is also available in supplements; however, before getting alarmed check with your doctor to see if you have a deficiency.

UPSIDES OF AGING: Sorry I didn't realize there was an upside to aging but as I experience every day and realize it is inevitable, I really enjoyed this information that makes some good points on the positives of aging. For many elders, it says, life past seventy is better than they imagined it to be. It's filled with challenges but lots of new horizons. Here are some points that were given by a noted gerontologist: ATTITUDE-If your attitude is that you're still good, you still enjoy life, there's still purpose in your life, you'll do well.

GREER POINT-now the secret to this is to position yourself where you can feel this way. If you hang around aging people who do not feel this way you are doomed. You must figure out a way to stay in the "main stream" of life, and that is easier said than done for many.

EMBRACE THE OPPORTUNITIES-Each decade and each age has opportunities that weren't actually there in the previous time. There have been joys in each stage of life. The thing is, people are so afraid of getting old. Don't worry about it. It's an adventure.

GREER POINT-couldn't agree more with these statements; however, the key to having this feeling and attitude is maintaining good health. So, nutrition and exercise are a key ingredient to being able to maintain a good attitude. Your health is your true wealth!!!

YOU HAVE SAGE ADVICE TO GIVE-As experienced people of this world, part of the aging process should be the ability to share this with younger people. As you age you gather knowledge and experience that should be worthwhile to the younger generation.

GREER POINT-While the accumulation of knowledge and experience is correct the ability to share it with the young is more challenging than one might think. Depending on the culture you are in determines how much you can really share. In the culture I happen to be in, which is the one I know the most about, the young do not have the same respect for the elderly. Sometimes they feel you are in their way to success or they do not have the patience to sit back and listen.

With the new electronic means of communicating it has changed our world to instant and continuous communication that many times leads to not getting things done.

When I go out to dinner with people in the twenty-five to forty age groups, I find the first thing they do is pull out their cell phones and then they start texting. When I am out with people in my age group sixty-five to seventy-five you never see their cell phones since they communicate the old fashion way, with their minds and mouth.

The real key to healthy, happy aging is to feel good in the age that you currently are. Never wish to be younger but to be healthier as the years go by. Then you have the knowledge and experience to share this with whomever may want to listen.

Notes:

CHAPTER 3

Physical Exercise

Take care of your body, it's the only place you have to live.

—Jim Rohn

Physical Exercise: Most people that know me or have known me for some time have this weird assumption that I have always exercised and that it comes naturally with me and is not a chore. Well, that is totally correct and gives me some bonus points going in since I don't have to make myself do the exercise thing. I have always believed I have been blessed with this attribute since exercise of any form is very important to our lives. I know of people who think that people who exercise are somewhat on the freaky side of life. I had a friend a few years ago who said he thought I was insane to exercise and that he had searched all over Dallas to find a doctor that would tell him exercise was bad for you. So, he did, and exercise is not part of his life.

To me, that is too bad for him, but I do know he is in his eighties now, and I guess he has proved something on the subject of exercise. But in my case, I consider it part of my lifestyle and from this, I am blessed with good health and strength, and I believe it belongs in the Eleven Points! While I am considered a fanatic, I must confess that I do love the production of sweat when I exercise and the fatigue that I feel after a good workout is only equaled by the good feeling of sex. Since I do seem to exercise to extremes, sometimes I would like to clarify where I really stand on this subject. I know and believe that a person can be minimally fit (enough to make a difference in good health) by only exercising three to four days a week and doing some form of aerobic exercise.

This means that a person would only have to keep the heart rate up for twenty to thirty minutes, at seventy-five percent of maximum for their age. The creator of the word *aerobic* was Dr. Ken Cooper of the Cooper Clinic, Dallas, Texas. His plea with the populace was to exercise moderately enough to encourage your body to be healthy. He was so bold as to make the statement that if a person runs over three miles at any given time, they are running too much. He should know, since he had done some marathons early on, and they taught him the lesson of "Lesser is better!"

The other part of this exercise thing is that walking, jogging, or running are not the only ways to raise that heart rate and sustain it for twenty to thirty minutes. It works in swimming, bicycling, soccer, etc., just to mention a few. The main thing is to enjoy whatever exercise is chosen. What I found in long-distance running, like the 26.2 marathon, is the beating that the body takes during this time in some way defeats the purpose. But, on the other hand, if a person wants to be extremely fit and still compete in something, the competitive running as an age group amateur gives a person the opportunity to still compete and enjoy themselves.

When I started to burn out on the marathon running, I decided to switch to the sport of triathlon and have found that swimming, biking, and running are excellent ways to maintain and build longevity in the body. Cross-training is very good, and that is what triathlon does for you. In some instances where a person does not like to swim, they can do duathlons, which require biking and running. Regardless of what someone decides to do to stay fit, I always suggest moderation to start with, and only advance to longer distances and competition if there is a strong desire for this. It is my feeling that exercise also gives a person an excellent outlet to relieve tension and even anger. I have seen some very positive and productive things come out of a good exercise program.

During my US Army days, I had a fellow officer approach me on the question of how he could lose his extra weight by exercising. He was almost in a panic mode, since he was going to lose his officer commission if he did not lose weight and meet the Army weight standards. He decided that walking or jogging would be the most favorable approach for him. The next thing I told him to do was buy some good running shoes and jogging apparel, if he didn't already have them.

Since this guy had never been into any kind of exercise program, I had to start from scratch with him. My instructions to him were to put on the jogging outfit and make himself go outside three days a week. Even if he didn't want to walk or jog right off, still just go outside and sit on the curb for twenty minutes. The good news is he did start jogging after his second time outside, and he even increased it by twenty more minutes after about a week. The good news is he started to enjoy how he felt and by the same token, he lost the excess weight within six weeks, and he was really proud of this accomplishment. So,

I believe there is a real need for all the population to have some form of exercise program, and I am proud to say I love it!

To further emphasize what I have defined as "moderation fitness for optimum health," I would like to share some of the fitness activities from Dr. Weil. He says it is probably possible to lead an inactive life and still experience healthy aging, *but not likely!*

Almost all the seniors he knows are very active, and they dance, walk, swim, cycle, golf, do yoga and tai chi. Of course, there are those still doing endurance sports way up into their seventies and some even into their eighties.

But this is a small portion and the moderation fitness mode is still highly recommended by most fitness gurus. Dr. Weil also emphasizes that it is possible to get too much physical activity, not just because over activity raises the possibility of damaging joints, muscles, and bones but also because of possible adverse effects on body composition, the nervous system, and reproductive and immune function.

He is a big advocate of walking, swimming, cycling, exercise machine workouts, and strength training. This follows my recommendation of moderation fitness and aerobic training. As I look at my life and the fact that I am in the category of an elderly person at seventy-six, I truly understand what he is saying. Even though I have trained for years to do marathons and Ironman triathlons, I now recognize this thing called aging. So what compulsive-lifestyle people like me do is adjust all our training and competing to match our level of aging and our body capabilities for our age. This past week, I finished some rehab work on my right fractured ankle (my eight-hundred-pound motorcycle fell on me) and I learned that my return to full triathlon training was affected by this injury.

But the good news is due to my healthy fitness practices over the years, my body recovered from this injury in the same time frame as a young adult's.

My physical therapist told me this after my boot was removed. But, on the other hand, I have also learned that I have diminished in some of my athletic strength, so I must adjust for that in my training and competition. Even though I have done seven Ironman Triathlons and twenty-five half Ironman events, I am cutting my participation back in these distances, but still competing in swimming, biking, and running events that are much shorter in distance. So, my training is also less to accommodate that, plus I have the opportunity to still compete. In triathlon, the age-group divisions go up to ninety to ninety-five (I have a friend in California who is still competing at ninety-one). Bottom line here is I emphasize that while I am a strong believer in exercise, I also know many people just do not want to spend their time sweating!

Just for grins, here are some of the excuses for not exercising that I have heard over the years: I don't have enough time for it (classic excuse, and I emphasize here that the aerobic exercise I recommend is thirty to forty-five minutes, three times per week, raising your heart rate very moderately). Anyone can spend this much time if they really want to. One way to do this is to not name this time exercising but maybe call it self-gratification time!

Next on the list is I'm too old to start (the answer is, do what you can do and not go over board). Then there is I don't know how (what a lousy excuse with all we have before us now on the subject! As the commercial says, "Just Do It!") Then last but not least—I just don't like it (this excuse will probably always win in the end and possibly, unless there is a life-threatening event, keep a person away from exercising).

But I have seen people who have heart attacks and then open-heart surgery who live through it, and *then* they decide they better do something or else they will be gone. My advice runs hand in hand with Dr. Weil's and I *never* try to talk anyone into endurance-type training, but I always emphasize the moderation fitness theme. When I have people who come to me wanting to find out how they start triathloning, I have a system that teaches them how to gradually enter this sport. Since it is a stair-step method of trying it out before a big commitment, I have found it always works.

What I tell people who have never done a triathlon and would like to is this: Get a bicycle, a place to swim and run, and do each discipline for the next three weeks, three times per week for thirty minutes. After this three-week period, I tell them if they are still interested, then they should up their time to forty-five minutes for each discipline for three weeks. Then if they are still interested, I tell them to up their time to sixty minutes. By the time they have done this for nine weeks and then come back to me for my advice, I recommend they get themselves a basic triathlon coach and go for it. If they never come back, then I know they either didn't want to do what I asked, or they didn't like triathlons as much as they thought they would.

Exercise should be fun if possible, but still enough to get that heart rate up there to help build strength in it. While many body builders will spend endless hours in the gym making their muscles look big and bulky, I feel like this is a big waste unless they are doing some cardio. Most cross-fit training (which is very good) and body building do not have enough cardio. So,

I really believe that longevity and healthy ageless living happens when you get good aerobic exercise,

"Snort, Spit and Blow, Movie Reviews" 3.28.2012

Running has for sure become a social thing more than a running thing. Not that this is all bad since it does get people off the couch and out the door. This past weekend I took some big-time mental notes of what was going on prior, during and after the 15,000-person Rock N Roll half marathon in Big D Texas. Since I was there for the running portion, I like to get to the start line early for warm up and stretching so I took note of this "new era" runner.

First, they really like to socialize before the event and spend a lot of time comparing notes on the latest running outfits, pre-race eating and drinking, and just useless gab that has nothing to do with why we are there. Again, not a bad thing just a different thing for us old timers who helped start this boom back in the stone ages. We used to get to the start line warmed up, juiced up and ready to run as fast as the body would allow. No discussion, just run like hell and get out of my way.

Now the events have a lot of walkers in them and I think that is a good thing since it pads the number of entry fees and helps pay for the event, plus "they" are doing something instead of nothing. Also, I notice the female population has really increased their running participation and that is a good thing, especially if they are good looking. Sorry, but my selfishness for taking my mind off the running pain centers due to looking at good looking women as they run. When it comes to this, I do not mind the fashion, running bra and all!! Ooops back to the subject at hand!

The actual running of the event gives the more experienced runners (in other words the old timers) a chance to get with it and see how fast the motor is for the day. Some of my running friends from the past used to tell me that running with me was like running with a horse, since I snort a lot, spit a lot and blow my nose as I run. The spitting came from many years on the football turf, since footballers spit a lot, and we had real grass and dirt to spit on. I try to avoid hitting some other runners with it but with 15,000 how do you have enough space? The snorting is no problem, just goes with the sound of running.

Then there is the nose blowing, something that just comes naturally for me when I run. I use the "put my thumb" on the opposite nostril that I am blowing from (a man thing, since I never see a woman blow their nose that way) method and it causes a projectile of snot that can annoy others I am sure. But this is a runner's prerogative and I do my best not to hit someone else, but again with a sea of runners how do you have enough space. During this last race I know I hit a few people with it, but they didn't seem to care. If a runner looks like they are in my age group, I try to hit right before they take a step so they might slip a little and give me an edge in placing higher in the age group. The problem with that is my age group is that "old" group I mentioned, and they are very clever about avoiding any kind of contact. With the spitting there is a little more control and not near as many people get hit by my spit bombs. Warning, don't bug me when I am running!

"Positives and Negatives of Being an Athlete" 8.26.2007

My earliest memory in my life involved a form of athletics. While doing a life time regression chart I was asked to go back as far as possible and recall my first memory.

Well it turned out that my first memory, that I could possibly recall, was running through a park in Pampa, Texas when I was two years old. My mother confirmed this age and remembered it well, since she said all I would do is run, run, run. So, I am sure she became weary of having to contain me or chase me, but regardless she had vivid memories of this.

While the race has all forms of activities going on in it the newer races now have live bands and lots of activities taking place during the race. Again, a very social atmosphere! While this is fine and dandy it also takes away from why we are there. I am not there to hear the latest hot tune or to even sing along with the music or talk about the latest fashions,

I am there, by God, to run, snort, spit, blow my nose, sweat, hurt, de-hydrate, ache, cramp, and generally feel very bad at the end. This is simply because that is what this thing called "running and racing" is all about. It is called a "good feel, bad feeling!" A way of life or possibly a life style! Who cares just get out of my way, my left hand is moving to my left nostril, beware!!

Now as I go through the memory jog of my life, I see that some form of athletics has always been in my life, so society puts me in the category of an "athlete." Whether it be team sports, or individual sports I am there and all over it. Being an athlete has given me an opportunity to put my God given talents to use either in competitive team sports or some individual sports that I like. It has been fun to compete in something athletically since I was 10 years old and then to still be competing in something fifty-eight years later.

That again would be the beautiful part of the sport of triathlon, in that you can still compete, no matter the age, and be welcomed into the field of competition just like the overall winners.

So, with, I would say I am thankful to be called an athlete and have enjoyed it for some time. The many positives of this designation are way too many to mention but I must mention a few so I can make my point in this writing. Being an athlete means, generally, that you will put your body to use in the field of competition with it being well trained and conditioned to compete at the highest possible level, no matter the sport.

This also means that as an athlete one would put out the maximum effort possible to prepare for the ultimate test of competition. During that preparation, depending on the sport, there may be pain, injury, sickness, depression, poor weather, poor coaching, poor attitude, etc. But regardless of these negatives the athlete pushes on and achieves his/her goal of competing to the utmost.

On the positive side the athlete is doing something they enjoy, is being recognized as an athlete and in many societies an actual hero and is whistling along on their merry way enjoying life.

In the community the athlete is generally put a notch above the non-athlete (not necessarily an attitude I agree with) and again is considered some kind of hero. On the same token the athlete thing starts to acquire that "swagger" that puts them apart from the other slugs in our society.

The prime example is the swagger referred to when talking about football quarterbacks. They are also called "field generals" and really have or acquire that special swagger only reserved for them. So, now maybe we have a bird's eye view of this thing called an athlete and what makes them feel so special or even over rates their attitude about their position way above where it really should be in life. Now this attitude and appearance turns to a thing called arrogance, cockiness, etc. Then the only thing that can really knock this down is failure to perform, or just not living up to the standards set by our loving society and then being abandoned by them.

The other major thing that can come along and wake the athlete up is a thing called, diminishing physical abilities caused by natural aging or major illness. When this happens, it makes the playing field altogether equal, and now it is time to survive.

This is also bringing my writing to the main point of typing today, many times the athlete will use his/ her trained mindset to ignore the pain of illness or simply ignore some tell-tale symptoms that cannot be ignored and must be addressed. A famous slogan among athletes is, "no pain, no gain."

Well what I have learned about accepting the pain thrust upon me by my infamous abscessed tooth and ignoring it for nearly three months, is that this pain I endured was getting one step closer to some very serious health problems or even a visit from the grim reaper.

So, now I have learned another valuable lesson in life by being the tough guy and working through pain, or even ignoring it, is not a good thing. Since this is some form of warning from the body of something being wrong, it should be addressed and taken care of. My plea to all athletes out there in competition land, is wake up and listen because your body maybe trying to tell you something that will be of benefit to your health in the future. Daily I have someone say, "you sure don't look your age, or you are so healthy, etc." While I am thankful people would say these things, I wonder what they would say if I conked over a stupid abscessed tooth. Boy, they would say, "what a waste, all he had to do was go to the dentist and get it removed, guess his athletic ego got in the way and he just wanted to work through the pain, and it would go away." Regardless, I hope my loyal readers get my point and now I promise in the future to get back to something with humor in it.

While our baseball little leaguers didn't win the World Series yesterday, they did win the hearts and minds of this community and the other people they met. They offered some humorous tidbits in their interviews. When asked by ESPN if they thought Coach Knight would win a National Championship in Texas Tech Basketball, one answered, "I think he can, he works them hard enough, and if they don't do what he says, he throws something at them!!"

Notes:

CHAPTER 4

Mental Exercise

Tell me and I forget, teach me and I remember, involve me and I learn.

—Benjamin Franklin

Mental Exercise: Now, to team up the mind with the body is really an important aspect of healthy aging. However, I would like to point out when the body is active, the mind will just follow along with it and make a great dancing-through-life partner. I have found that when I do aerobic exercise, my mind tends to go into high gear and really produce some thought-provoking subjects. While there are different aspects that go on in the mind, I would say that the main topics would be spiritual, creative, reactive, visual, negative or positive thoughts, sadness, happiness, fear, etc.

Philosopher Kierkegaard stated: "To live only in necessity is to live as if I am what I am and can be no different. To live only in possibility is to live as if I can be whatever I imagine. Life's greatest tragedies are to be found in people who have cared too much (or too little), or who have willed too much (or too little). It takes inner strength and wisdom to recognize and accept our own limitations, but only by going through this process will we become able to transcend them."

A few years ago, I worked with a very creative business consultant, and after she had done a study on my manufacturing business, she gave me the final report. But I think one of the most important things she said in the concluding meeting was that I must always be true to myself. Fact is she wrote that out on a piece of paper and taped it to my Day Timer, which I kept for a long time. If we are not true to ourselves, we more than likely cannot be true to others, plus this gives us a great entrée into the golden years. That way, there is no regret and no remorse.

Mental exercise can consist of several things that put our minds to work but doesn't create headaches. If I try to do crossword puzzles, it gives me a headache, so I stay away from that mind activity. While reading is one of the things that I have developed over the years, I have found that my personal library is very diverse with lots of different subjects. I do not read fiction simply because I want to read about actual people or real activities.

As I look on my bookshelf, I find such diversity as George Carlin (a weird brand of humor). John Maxwell (excellent leadership, management, self-help, subjects with a creative way to present them), Mike Leach (college football coach with a sense of humor and odd subjects, but not about football), Bobby Knight (college Hall of Fame basketball coach), Billy Crystal (humor), Howard Buffet (how to feed the starving children of the world), Elizabeth Warren (US senator), and last but not least, the King James Version of the Bible, to name a few of my four-hundred-book library.

Another form of mental exercise that I have adopted is the study of the American presidents. While I have never been a real history buff, I have found that as I study these guys, I find that I learn a lot of American history. But my focus is on them while reading about their service to the country. Most of my references have complete details of the presidents and it is enjoyable to read about their accomplishments and what made them different from each other.

This hobby has been a great exercise for my mind, and as I enter into a conversation on the subject, I find my mind searching for certain answers to the questions that are brought up during the conversation. My trips to Washington, DC, are more meaningful now as I see the different tributes to our nation's leaders. While there are many other things that we can do to exercise the mind, I think it is one of the most important aspects of life. But as I watched my father get all his ailments repaired, I saw his inactivity mentally completely speed up his aging. So, as part of my eleven points, I do want to mention balance as many times as I can because it is very important.

In 2005, I decided to enter the blogosphere for expressing myself. At first, I created the blog site www. fasttwitchmind.blogspot.com for the purpose of expressing off the wall or out of the blue opinions on life's many subjects. While I very seldom went over five hundred, I did exceed that at some point. Then a few years later, I created the www. maturefitness.blogspot.com site, dealing specifically in fitness-related topics. By having these two topics, I can venture into general life's subjects and then get specific with the *Mature Fitness* blog. On the Fast Twitch Mind blog, I will sometimes just ask for a random word from friends and then create a blog from that one word, or I will be driving down the road and think of what I think is a good subject, then I start writing about it when I get to my office.

The purpose for these two sites is not to change the world but to keep my mind working and creating and that I believe will take me into my nineties. While I try to stay on the positive side, or at least with a strong sense of humor, sometimes the negatives will creep in and then I must pull out the mental eraser! It is very important to neutralize negative images by constantly calling upon positive ones. George Lakoff, a professor of cognitive science and linguistics at the University of California, Berkeley, has written about his experience of the terrorist attacks on the World Trade Center on September 11, 2001, in his insightful book, *Don't Think of an Elephant!* He says, "I now realize that the image of the plane going into South Tower was for me an image of a bullet going through someone's head, the flames pouring from the other side like blood spurting out. It was an assassination. The tower falling was a body falling. The image afterward was hell: ashes, smoke and steam rising, the building skeleton, darkness, suffering, death…By day the consequences flooded my mind; by night the images had me breathing heavily, nightmares. keeping me awake. Those symbols lived in the emotional centers of my brain."

As I have aged, I have experienced the passing of my parents and only sibling before their time, and I find myself thinking of them frequently. Most of my thoughts are positive, but the advice I would give people, if asked, is if there is some form of estrangement in the family, I would try to get it resolved, since it will be impossible to do after they are gone. Only the potential memory of what it would be like is what will be in the mind. As the aging process sets in, it is important to stay active mentally and always have some kind of activity going on.

Here are some good thoughts from Dr. Weil: Learn to identify habitual thoughts and images that produce feelings of sadness or anxiety, particularly those about the process of aging and changes in your body and appearance. He also says that we should not try to stop negative thinking or imagery. Instead, practice substituting positive thoughts and images that evoke feelings of happiness and security.

It takes practice to change mental habits. Just keep at it!

"Memory Loss" 5.8.2011

A few days ago, I came to the reality that memory loss is not associated with age. As I walked out of the aquatic center and couldn't remember where I had parked my car, I was sure I was losing it. Then I got to thinking that memory loss starts very early in life and in fact is not associated with age. For example, I have no memory of the day I was born. But I know it happened for several reasons, i.e. I am here today, my birth certificate says I was born, and every year I celebrate my birthday on December sixteenth.

But, back to the location of my Explorer somewhere in the parking lot. As I wondered through the maze of SUV's I became totally aware that there is short term (where the hell is my Explorer) and long-term loss, like someone reminds you of something you did when you were a teenager and you have no memory of that. Good news, memory loss is not fatal.

"Spelled Out" 9.2010

A few times I have probably mentioned that life has become just way too complicated and everything seems to revolve around the computer, iPhone, e-mail, text-mail, twitter, twatter, Facebook, in-your face, and all that garbage. That is not to mention the fax machine, which still exists, typewriter (which doesn't exist that I know of), ball point pen, #2 pencil, and smoke signals.

Well there is another method of communicating that has now become sort of complicated, it is called talking to your pets by having to spell words so as not to upset them or get them all hyper. Buffman & Squeaky have reached that mentality that is driving me nuts.

While the Boston Terrier is one smart breed of dogs ol' Buffman (nine years), and Squeaky (four years) have now exceeded that by learning the English language to such a point that we are now having to spell things out, so they do not get too excited about what is fixing to happen. Case in point, if we happen to slip and say we are going somewhere (which doesn't matter where, just saying GO OR GOING seems to be the key word) then they start barking, jumping, chewing, and grabbing the leash so they can GO. Then if they are not going, we must go through the explanations of why they are not going and then give them a cookie (dog bone).

The bad part about this is they could be conning us to get the cookie, but on the other hand we always give them one when we leave without them. So, now we have started spelling everything.

So, we can't use the words, running, walking, going, playing, riding the motorcycle, going to town, going to a movie, without spelling it out. Right now, that is working but it will not be long before they figure it out. Oh, I forgot, you can't open the drawer where the leashes are unless you want two Boston terriers licking and leaping all over your legs raving to GO!! I am thinking the next step might be sign language, but by some of the expressions on Buff's face I know he will figure that one out quick. This dog can look at you with the most, "what in the hell is this human thinking?" expressions I have ever seen.

In the mornings he will give me his good morning look by standing on the arm of the chair over my lap, turns his head for a slight minute staring right into my eyes. He then turns his head the other way, and steps down. Like, well I have done my duty to this dude called master, and now to get on with my day of sleeping, barking, pooping, peeing, eating, and licking. On the other hand, Squeaky just looks at me with a dead pan look of, "why bother?" I am going to just do my thing, sleep, bark, poop, pee, eat and lick when I want to. For me, I will GO (spelled out) and DO (spelled out) my thing for the day, wondering what challenges they have in store for me upon my return.

MIKE GREER, PhD.

Notes:

CHAPTER 5

Active Social/Sex Life

Love is like a virus. It can happen to anybody at any time.

—Maya Angelou

Active Sex (Social) Life: While I have enjoyed talking about the first four points, I must say I am glad to get to number five. As I present this point to live groups, I always wonder how it is going to be taken or perceived; however, I always emphasize that one size does not always fit all and these are *my* eleven points, and the subject of an active sex life has always been very important to me. Now, also please note the wording in the title is Active Sex (Social) Life. The reason for that is I do make and have made this presentation to age groups down to fourteen to seventeen, and I am sure that suggesting an active sex life to this age group would not be a smart move. So, I change this to Active Social Life when I am presenting to young groups.

With that being said, I would like to venture into this subject with open eyes and an open mind. Since it is a fact of life that the "facts" of life are a very big part of our adult lives. As I consult with the King James Version of the Bible, I find that immediately after God created the Earth, he created man and woman. It wasn't long before they figured out their nakedness and then they "knew" each other, and the first generation of children were born. While I know the story has more details, it is basically as I described it and regardless of how one believes about the story in the Holy Bible, it really doesn't matter, since "knowing" and "having sex" is all part of the creation of the world. With that being said, let's move on to the modern world and how our sex life affects us and what it means to us. Whether we talk procreation sex or just enjoyment sex, it doesn't matter since both are very important to our lives. Again, we can probably have some great debates over this, but for now I will stick to my point and move on.

Napoleon Hill, author of *Think and Grow Rich,* wrote this book in 1960, and it has been in my library since 1970. While I have enjoyed the book and have referenced it on many occasions, I have always felt it was mistitled simply because it is just not about making money and being rich, it is about knowing life and being rich in all things, such as education, ethics, sharing, etc. Fact is, I adopted a theme early in my life that was influenced by this book in that I have always felt I am very wealthy if I have excellent health.

Along with this belief and practice I have always felt that as long as I can do whatever I want, I am also wealthy. Now along the way, this book has also enhanced my abilities to make more income than I need, but it also gave me tremendous advice when I needed it. While I am not pushing this book to make some money off it, I would say that it is preeminently a "what-to-do and how-to-do-it" book. In it, you will find the magic of self-direction, organized planning, and auto-suggestion, mastermind association, and an amazingly revealing system of self-analysis. Now in this little old book there are some great thoughts about an active and healthy sex life. While it must be understood that Mr. Hill is not a psychologist, marriage counselor, sex therapist, or life coach, he is a guy that has done tremendous research in all phases of life for the opportunity to offer solid advice to mankind on how to be successful in all walks of life. So, he says that the sex desire is the most powerful of human desires.

The emotion of sex brings into being a state of mind. When driven by this desire, men develop keenness of imagination, courage, willpower, and creative ability unknown to them at other times. So strong and compelling is the desire for sexual contact, that men freely run the risk of life and reputation to indulge in it. Many men of extreme wealth and power have given it all up for the opportunity to be with a certain woman. In considering the ten stimuli of the mind, he lists "the desire for sex expression" as number one.

With that being said, I do not want to overemphasize the fifth point of my eleven, but, on the other hand, the points made by Mr. Hill are very good and needed to be said by someone. As I discovered my sexual feelings very early in life, I have to say I agree with his assessments one hundred percent and look forward to number five for the rest of my life. While I realize I have not ventured into the many details associated with this activity of life, I really do not think it is necessary. For example, I am sure that within some deep intellectual discussions about this subject, the group would want to know in detail what makes an active sex life, and does it vary or change when we age. Well, I think the answer to this lies within the individual and the frequency of the sexual act really rests with the individual. Now does the frequency of sex diminish with age, probably more yes than no. But the thoughts and desires may still be there, but the aging body and mind might not be as willing.

In *Healthy Aging,* Dr. Weil discusses the aging sexual life very well and while he wrote twenty-one pages describing the anti-inflammatory diet as opposed to three pages on touching and sex, I believe he is being very realistic on what he does say. He does state that sexuality changes as you grow older. He also offers some strategies to make peace with changes in your sexual life.

1. Get good medical advice if needed
2. Have open communication with your partner
3. Use all sources to find an appropriate partner
4. Self-stimulation is always an option
5. *Remember everyone is different!*

There are no set rules. Pay attention to how your interests and appetites change. *Get the book!* It is worth the money!

"The Conductor" 3.5.201

How can something the size of a walnut have so much power over a healthy life style and have the gall to interfere with a good night's sleep or an active sex life? Well let me tell you folks out there that little dude has received a special name and designation from me, and I am proud to share it.

The prostate gland sits in such a cozy little place in the human body that it has tremendous influence on what goes on regarding sexual activity and passing of the urine that I have re-named it "The Conductor."

The conductor on the passenger trains used to be the person who made everything happen for its passengers and even gave the green light for the train to start moving. He was always a "he," but had on those snappy little black suits, white shirt, and a black bow tie.

Now I am not proposing the little walnut that sits down there all decked out in black, but you know it wouldn't surprise me if it is.

The conductor of the male body sits at such a strategic point that it has a strangle hold on the urethra and can affect the bladder in very negative ways. Since the urethra itself has some fairly large duties and prides itself in being able to pass semen and urine to the respective outlets it becomes very irritated when ole bully walnut squeezes it off and won't let it function properly. It has been nicknamed the "Double Teamer," by those in the know. So, then the captain of the ship (human male body person) gets really irritated when the sex life and passing of urine does not happen as it should. Also, not to mention having to pass urine in the worst possible time or the opposite of not being able to pass urine at the most opportune time.

Since all males over the age of about sixty (give or take a few years per individual) start to experience the possible difficulties with the conductor, my purpose here is to shout out and let you know that this is all very normal.

The walnut gland is the only gland that continues to grow in the body, so the longer we live the larger it gets.

Now to take control of the Mr. Fatty Conductor there are options starting with drugs that shrink it (with side effects most of us do not want, i.e. it affects our sex life, so then we have to take other drugs to offset that) or the old roto rooter method of shaving the excess fat off with a metal shaving device, which causes some side effects, long recovery, and lots of bleeding.

Now comes along the modern-day treatment of reducing the walnut with a laser treatment that is a one-hour procedure, recovery is much quicker, blood loss much less, and should be good for seven years. With acronym names such as, TURP, Green Light, and HoLap, sounds like fun to me!

Now as the "Conductor" says, "all aboard Mr. Laserman, take charge and go after that dude that has gone from walnut size to small apple size!" Note: Is that where the term, "not comparing apples to apples came from?"

"Little Walnut" 1.18.2014

It appears every time I go to the mail box there is another mailer out concerning the prostate gland or the brain. What one has to do with the other is beyond me, but I do know they are hot subjects. The prostate (little walnut) is popular now because it basically came out of the closet of silence since only men have them, and they weren't exactly keen about talking about this little critter until now. Well why not make it a hot subject since the minute the urologist withdraws his 3"x 7" index finger the fun begins.

Maybe in the next edition I will cover some of the gritty details, but now I want to move to the brain. It is funny how different the doctors are in each specialty.

Here we have a person (usually male) who likes to check things out from the rear side to the neurologist who checks out the brain waves that make us do what we do or don't do. But I do know I have much more experience with the urologist than the brain docs. Does that mean I have more prostate than brain, well possibly but thankfully I have only had to visit the brain guy one time.

While it is common to have an enlarged prostate at age seventy, I am convinced that the brain shrinks by the time we are seventy. It seems so unfair since we really need all the brain power we can get just to move through the day. In addition to receiving literature that tells me how to shrink my prostate, have better sex and more importantly have a smooth urine flow, I also get tons of mail about exercising and saving the brain.

There seems to be thousands of lists from one to ten, or things to do to preserve the brain and improve its functions. The other day I saw a magazine that told how to keep your brain active and healthy. It said that going to movies was very healthy and reduced stress, since you go into a darkened movie theater with elevated comfort seats and enjoy the entertainment of a great movie. Of course, it didn't cover what happens to the nervous system when you see gory blood slinging gangster or horror movies. At any rate, possibly I have touched on two hot subjects and now I would like to cover my current movie adventures.

"Birds and the Bees" 11.8.2009

The birds and the bee's expression has been around since the beginning of time, as far as I know. I am guessing that it really became a point of conversation after Adam, in all his naked glory, took that infamous bite of the forbidden fruit. While he was crunching on the juicy delicious shiny red apple, he looked down south and discovered the tools of the trade that would soon get him in deep trouble. Along these same lines I suppose he came up with that quaint little expression, while conversing with Eve about reproduction and other sexual topics, "the birds and the bees."

While I have only been on this earth a relatively short time compared to the overall big picture of creation, I have always heard this expression when it comes to discussing sex and other related subjects. For the life of me I do understand the bee's role in this drama, and I am not sure what the birds have to do with it either. I would think the expression "rabbits and bees" would better describe reproduction than "birds and bees." The male rabbit is well known for his abundance of testosterone and the female rabbit is equally proud of her ability to conceive and produce many offspring.

But before I go on the crusade to change this expression, I want to convey my recent experience with a bee and how he showed me how it got the reputation of a reproducer. I was laying out in the backyard gathering up some unusual November sun and was drinking a coke out of a can.

As I sat up and put the can between my legs, this bee approached me. I sat there very calm and watched it do its little bee thing of going around in rapid circles, moving its wings at one hundred RPMs, and sighting on the best possible place he could land to start gathering this sweet sugar, then taking it home to the hive to reproduce and make a little honey. It was interesting to watch the bee make the circle, then make the approach and then the landing.

As he started nuzzling the coke at the top of the can he decided to go inside the can. When he went down inside, he must have gotten a real strong taste of sugar and caffeine, since he was a tad bit wobbly and had a little trouble initiating the flight off the can. Again, I just sat there with patience and no fear that he would sting me.

He then started flying again, made a couple of passes and then made another landing. He looked at me like, hey dude this is good stuff and I want a little more. He then went back inside the can, guzzled some more coke, came back out and then flew off to the mother land. Now I understand the "birds and the bees" expression a little better, but I still believe the rabbit has a place in this story. In this modern world of electronics, I sometimes get very frustrated and wonder what happened to some of the simple words that were used to help you operate these gadgets.

To best illustrate my point, I think the most important thing you need to know is where the "off" and "on" buttons are on things that are powered by whatever means. But I have noticed these two words are used less and less each time something is manufactured. When I go to turn the television on, I want to just look for the on button and simply turn it on. But now we have three different hand-held control gadgets that do not have on or off on either of them.

They have words like, power (probably on, but a guess), select (that is if you get it turned on), recall (recall what if you can't turn it on), play, stop (stop what, if I can't get the damn thing on), mute, search, pause, and browse (Again all of this is moot if you can't turn it on). Then there is the computer, no off and on anywhere, but you do have enter, shift, backspace, num lock, control, tab, home, caps lock, end, page up, page down, etc., but no off and on. I have discovered a black button on the main face of the computer box that does allow me to shut this thing off if I get really frustrated.

The other day it just froze, so I defrosted it by hitting this button that didn't say "off." Fact is, it doesn't say anything. Then there are cell phones that have talk, end, back, text, next, space, but no "off" and "on." We have a couple of those little electric heaters for the exercise room and they do not have "off" and "on" buttons. But they do have mode, osc, timer so I just start hitting buttons until something happens that I like and be done with it.

After searching all over the house for something with "off" and "on" on it I finally found it with my alarm clock. Believe it or not it was off, on, buzzer, alarm, dream bar, snooze and sleep. So, there is hope that maybe these two words will return to power objects and mankind will not have to be left guessing.

This morning someone sent me a very disturbing You Tube presentation of President Obama proclaiming he is a Muslim and that the United States is not a Christian nation. He proclaimed the goodness of Islam and covered in detail all the great things the Muslims have done for the United States. He even did something that no American president has ever done (including the oil loving W. man); he bowed to a Muslim hierarchy. Now I don't know where all these things come from, but I do know I have never seen as much stuff written about a president as there has been about his one. I even got one e-mail that had he and Mrs. Big O going to a costume party with him in a Joker costume and she in a very revealing (at least D cups) costume with the belly button showing. When I am asked, what are we going to do about this president?

My only response is—get your butt off the couch at election time and vote him out of office. That is how we do things in this democracy and he became a master at raising money for the election (a record $745 million) and THEN getting the people to vote for him on Election Day.

They just didn't raise money for him; they also went out and voted for him. My thinking is that if all the Seniors (over sixty-five) in the country (approximately fifty-one million from what I can gather) went out and voted in the next election for the opposition candidate against President O, then there would be a chance for him to be defeated. Since ninety-five percent of the black voters in the country voted for him the senior population, with the same turn out, could get the job done. Come on Seniors, let's get out there and get it done.

Notes:

CHAPTER 6

Balance in Life

In the end it's not the years in your life that count. It's the life in your years.

—Abraham Lincoln

Balance in Life: While this point is easy to say, it is much harder to practice in the real world. While the word *moderation* is used here, that also is a very hard practice in reality, and there is the question of what moderation is and what does it mean. Depending on the culture we are born, raised, and live in, moderation will have many definitions and many practices.

In American culture, we are raised to basically be hard-driving people, goal setters, goal achievers, and reset the new goals after old goals are accomplished. So how do we live a balanced life and enjoy it? In my life coaching practice, the first thing that usually comes up are these statements from the client, "I feel like my life is so unbalanced, and I can't seem to get it on the right track!" or, "It is either so busy on one thing that three other things go bad, so how do I get the balance I need?"

At this point, I would say that this client's life is out of balance, and there are certain steps that can be taken to get it more balanced and keep it balanced. In many cases, life gets out of control because of control dramas that come into play by those we are around during the waking hours. For example, if we are married, there is always the chance of control dramas by the spouse, and if there are children, then the same can happen. Then, in extremes, we have the relatives by marriage.

Since this is only one example of life-balancing negatives, it should also be pointed out that the profession, health, education, income, fun, etc., can stand in the way of life balance. What I recommend my clients to do is to sit down in a quiet room and complete the "wheel of life exercise" and determine what is happening that creates this lack of balance. My clients have used this method very effectively and it always illustrates, in black and white, what is going on. It is important to be very honest on this assessment and then plan after that.

I also know as we age, our balance of life activities can change, or will change. Again, the main thing is to maintain as much balance as possible and back off whatever might be hindering this. During my endurance training requirements, while getting ready for a long-distance event, I have found it always impairs the balance-of-life goal and getting back to normal must also be a goal once the event is concluded.

It will be my challenge to anyone reading this book to make a copy of the wheel of life exercise, and the daily habits list. Study these very closely, make the plan, and then implement the plan. It will only make you happier and relieve that claustrophobic feeling of everything closing in on you.

When speaking of balance in life, I believe the ego should be mentioned here. While I have debated about this within myself, I came away from my last discussion with me with a strong feeling that, first ego must be discussed, *and* it should be under the balance of life category. When talking ego amongst the general public, I have found it is usually used in a negative way and very seldom mentioned as a positive.

I have searched for a definition of it by our fellow Webster, and he simply states, "The conscious self." Then he goes on to define *egocentric* as "self-centered" and then *egotism* as "excessive concentration on one's self." With that being said, I think my point of the ego being misunderstood or ill-defined does come possibly from the point of view that when the society, public, media, or whatever labels something, good or bad, it will normally prevail just out of habit.

When I think of ego, I like to think of an ego that drives a person to the point of ultimate achievement from the good side, then I think of the overgrown (like an overgrown toe nail) ego that drives a person to become controlling, dishonest, and obnoxious. In my opinion, there are good egos and bad egos and probably some just walking the line between both. But since I want to stay positive here, I would like to be so bold as to introduce a new definition or action statement relative to the *ego*. I believe strongly that if a person harvests the strengths of their ego, they can accomplish all the realistic goals they desire! It is also my feeling that by doing this, there will be much more balance in a person's life.

In the morning paper today, there was an interesting comment about egos that came from Pope Francis in one of his talks at a Vatican City conference. He was warning the new cardinals to keep the partying to a minimum—and keep their egos in check—when they are formally elevated at a Vatican ceremony next month. Wow, the word *ego* just got elevated, and I never dreamed it would be used in this context.

Please go back and review the previous paragraph about "harvesting the strengths of your ego so as to accomplish all of the realistic goals you desire!" Not saying my proclamation walks hand in hand with the pope's, but I really believe in the strength of our egos, in all walks of life. See the attached Wheel of Life exercise and Daily Habits list. It might include the following: your occupation, patterns of sleep, time for play and relaxation, time spent acquiring useful knowledge, and just plain wasting it! Remember, there are one-hundred-sixty-eight hours in a week.

"Ego" 1.24.2011

Ego is a simple three letter word that is used frequently throughout any given day. It is used to describe people that are all into themselves and then escalates to narcissism. I know, it sounds like a bad disease but really isn't. I have talked about the misuse of ego before on this blog but cannot recall everything I said so I was prompted to be reminded of this word again during the most recent inductee ceremonies of the USA Triathlon Hall of Fame, in Colorado Springs.

In 2004 when I was serving as the interim executive director of USA Triathlon, I suggested to the board that USAT should have their own Hall of Fame and it should be done on a very professional basis.

Even though the board drug their feet and moved it to a useless committee they finally moved it into the responsibility of a person that could get it done, and he did do that in a very professional way, using the good side of his ego.

So, in 2008 the Hall of Fame did become a reality and it has been my pleasure to attend the inductee ceremony on all three occasions.

As I listen to the introductions of the inductees and then I listen to their acceptance speeches the three-letter word "ego" comes to mind. Now you say, "hey wait a minute bub these guys and gals are the best of the best that the sport has to offer, in both the athletic and non-athletic side, so where are you coming from. Well first the word ego is not a bad word, it is simply defined by our old Webster as, "the self," "the rational part of the mind that controls actions." Now when you start throwing out, "egotism, egocentric, ego trip," it becomes another animal.

So, what I experienced on this Hall of Fame inductee night is a lot of ego but not on the negative side. It has always been my strong belief that a happy ego makes for a happy person, and a self-driven person, for the better. On the opposite side I see egos out of control that bring in the egotism, egocentric, and ego trip nature of the type of people who give the word a bad name. Throughout the acceptance speeches I heard the message of extreme pride in what they were doing and the inner drive to do what they were doing with a desire to do it to the best of their ability.

There was never the feeling that they were doing it all for themselves but shared the feeling of thanks and appreciation for all those who helped them achieve their successes.

It reminds me of the first time I was accused of having a big ego I asked the person who said it to illustrate my egotism.

After this person finished, I ask, "are you still driving your Lexus and do you still live in the trendy part of town with the finest furniture money can buy, and oops I forgot do your designer clothes still fit really good, etc., etc.?" Of course, I knew the answers to these innocent questions were all yes, I humbly mentioned that my vehicle of choice was a five-year-old SUV with over 100,000 miles on it, my place of residence at that time was in a nice neighborhood but certainly not trendy, etc.

So, who had the big ego here? In my opinion neither of us did, it was just a case of pointing out what ego is versus egotism, in a realistic comparison, and my point was well taken. It is so much fun to watch a healthy ego achieve so much in life. As I watch my professional friends achieve so much with their healthy egos, that lead to extreme successes and beyond reproach job satisfaction, it motivates me to do the same. I always encourage people to recognize this part of our personalities and use it to our best advantage. It works but can get out of control.

Notes:

CHAPTER 7

Transition through Life

It is only through labor and painful effort, by grim energy and resolute courage, that we move on to better things.

—Theodore Roosevelt

Passing through Life Transitions: This is probably one of the most forgotten aspects of living, aging, and acceptance. For example, the first time I wrote down these eleven points, there were only seven. Then, as I aged, I gained four more points to consider. So, the transitions of my life from age one to seventy-six have really existed and are still happening. I feel that the way we handle our transitions is the big influence on how our healthy ageless living becomes reality.

When we are younger, many of our transitions just happen very naturally and not much thinking is required; however, as we age, we must really make some decisions we may not want to make or face. While I realize that our health becomes a big factor in our aging, this only makes my points about healthy ageless living even more important to our lifestyle.

When I was in my forties, I went in for my annual physical exam, and at the conclusion of it, my doctor said, "Greer, you are going to be a lonely man when you are older!" I asked him why, and he said, "Because you are so healthy, all of your friends will be dead!" Then he laughed as he put the rubber glove on to give me that infamous index finger check on the little walnut called the prostate gland! Now, thirty-six years later, I am watching many of my friends pass away, just as the doctor said I would be.

So here I am, going through another of life's transitions, and I find it interesting and sometimes very frustrating, simply because I do not want to lose my good friends, and the other is I have found it impossible to replace those kinds of people. You can meet other people or go to new places, but you can never completely replace a best friend.

Now let's go back to when I was twenty-one and got married and went through that life transition. I will never forget it no matter how old I get. I recall making a pact with myself that I would always guard my thoughts and would never reveal *all* my thoughts or feelings. They would belong exclusively to me and would not be shared. To me this has been part of my ability to transition to another phase of my life more easily. I still have my private thoughts and will always practice that within myself. That is the same as my comfort food, music or conversation, my exercise, my competition, my business success—it is all mine.

The other aspect of passing through these transitions of life positively is I have found these times offer the opportunity to move out of our comfort zones and learn new things, establish new friendships, or have a completely new sense of accomplishment. The first time I traveled to Europe, I was by myself, did not speak German, and I took a passenger train from Southern Germany to the upper part of Northern

Germany. While I did not speak the language, I was able to navigate well on the train, figure out when to get on the train and when to get off, etc. So, I moved out of my comfort zone and felt more accomplished when I reached my destination.

I also recall when I left my job with a large company to start my own very small business. The movement out of the comfort zone at that time involved providing for a wife and four children, so moving out of my professional comfort zone was real and very motivating. Since I have been an athlete all my life, since the age of ten, I have also gone through transitions from one sport to another. Since we cannot play football all our lives, I transitioned into a sport called handball and played that for twelve years. Then, as I felt my body needing a change, I went to endurance running and triathlons.

Both sports gave me an opportunity to stay in good physical condition and compete in my current age group. After thirty-seven years of endurance competition, I find myself still longing for the training and competition, but on the other hand, I have learned with healthy aging, I can still train and compete, but I must do it with more control and respect for my body.

Again, another transition in life—making plan B my new plan A. As I mention plan B here in the positive tone, please do not interpret this to mean I design plan A with the thoughts that I will fail, so I automatically go into plan B. Sometimes, as we look at life and set goals, we must always consider them with the idea of accomplishment past where we are today. So that equates to accomplishment and not failure.

When I did my first Ironman, I had plans A, B, and C. The reason for this is because I had never done a 140.6-mile swim, bike, and run triathlon. At that time of the sport of triathlon, there was not an abundance of information on this distance. So,

I knew that some of this day would be devoted to "learning" and not really competing. I also wanted to finish this event in the required time (seventeen hours) so I would not have a DNF (did not finish) label on my running shorts. With that in mind, plan A was my optimum finish with the finish time I wanted at fourteen and a half hours standing up; plan B was a finish time of fifteen and a half hours, standing up; and then plan C with a finish time of sixteen and a half hours, standing up.

My actual finish time was sixteen hours and five minutes, standing up, and then spending some time in the medical tent taking in an IV. But my point here is that there were so many unknowns going into this event that I wanted to make sure I came out positive, and I did. We must realize that life transitions are very similar to this, and we must be willing to accept this as fact and then transition accordingly.

When I turned seventy, I decided to make me a new life-goal sheet, which had a little different make up and approach. On this goal sheet, I would draw a line across the sheet of white blank paper and put my current age of seventy on it. Then below this line, I would list all my lifetime accomplishments that had a major influence on my life, such as: educational, professional, spiritual, family, military, athletics, etc. Then I would draw two lines going upward, but not straight up. They would go at outward angles to the top of the page. This way, there would never be an ending and the new goal accomplishment section would be never ending. Please note the filled in goal sheet, and that one can be used by you to make your own infinite list of goals. When breaking through the transitions of life, always look at the finish of one and the beginning of the next as the opportunities to accomplish more positive things in life and continuing to build the legacy you leave.

"New Secrets to Living to 114" 4.17.2011

During the past week the oldest man in the world died at the age of one-hundred-fourteen. Walter Breuning of Great Falls, Montana said that his philosophies of life started when he was very young and his earliest memories stretched back 111 years, before home entertainment came with a twist of the radio dial. They were of his grandfather's tales of killing Southerners in the Civil War. Breuning was three and horrified: "I thought that was a hell of a thing to say." But the stories stuck and helped him to develop his own simple philosophies that guided him throughout his life.

Here are his secrets of a long life:

Embrace change, even when the change slaps you in the face, every change is good.

Eat two meals a day, that's all you need.

Work as long as you can, that money's going to come in handy.

Help others, the more you do for others, the better shape you're in.

Thanks, Mr. Breuning for the great example you set and for the exemplary words of wisdom.

Notes:

CHAPTER 8

Releasing Grudges

Forgive, forget, bear with the faults of others as you would have them bear with yours.

—Phillips Brooks

Prevent Holding Grudges: While this point was not in the original seven, I added it as a result of giving it some real hard thought. Again, remember I mentioned in the introduction about looking at the DNA of our parents to see what lifestyle practices they had that affected their health. Some of the practices of our parents would be obvious, such as lack of exercise, poor nutrition to the point of serious disease in their body, disturbing psychological attitudes, etc.

But there is one that I noticed in my dad's profile that I believe can really affect a healthy lifestyle. He was not able to forgive and forget other people when he had disagreements with them. He was for sure a grudge-holder, and I have read in many health journals that it is felt having these types of feelings over a long period of time can most certainly be a pathway to serious health problems.

My father had open-heart surgery, colon cancer, and prostate cancer. While surgery had corrected the heart problem, the colon cancer, and the prostate cancer, he still maintained his bad feelings with others he had had bad dealings with over the years. So, it has always been my feeling that we should do all we can to overcome holding grudges. Now it is a real dream world thing to think we would never have a disagreement or ill feelings with other people over our lifetime, but the secret is being able to release these feelings at some point.

In a real-life family and business dispute, I ended up with a disagreement with a relative that created terrible feelings within myself. So, while I still had the ill feelings toward the person, I knew in my mind I must relieve it at some time. In my heart and mind, I knew what had to happen for this to be and that is what I prayed for over the years.

The complication of it was for this to happen in the most possible way, the other person was going to have to take the initiative because of the circumstances of the incident. That is how I directed my prayers, and then twelve years later, I get a message from the other party stating that he wanted to come to Lubbock and buy me dinner and talk. So, I consented, and at this meeting he completely apologized to me for what he had done and said that he was very wrong in what happened, and he asked for my forgiveness. Since my prayers were answered, I was very thankful to God and to the offending person. We had a great dinner under very pleasant circumstances. I was completely relieved, and so was he!

Now that I have revealed a real-life incident covering this point, I would like to offer a step-by-step plan for preventing grudges in the first place, and then some possible action steps that can rid you from them. *Grudge* is defined as "resentment toward someone as a result of a major disagreement." I say major here because I cannot imagine anyone holding a long-term, health-threatening grudge over a small event in life. It is safe to say that whatever creates the grudge would have to be a major event in their life. I think of the legendary feud between the Hatfield's and McCoy's, which was major, and created many grudges between these two families. I would then say that a disagreement over whether a movie is a good movie or bad movie is not worth holding a grudge over. Obviously, the disagreeing parties I would think would have to decide when to end this disagreement, shake hands, and carry on with their lives.

The steps for clearing out the feeling of grudges should happen when:

1.   There is a recognition that the deep grudge does exist;
2.   There is a desire for this grudge to be relieved from both parties;
3.   There is a recommended remedy to eliminate these thoughts from both parties' minds;
4.   There is a willingness for both parties to meet and present the plan;
5.   There is agreement at the meeting, then the forgiveness and acceptance are acknowledged;
6.   Both parties truly *forgive* and *forget* the reason for the grudge and move on with their lives.

Many times in life, there is a high stress level that is brought on by the actions of those people that you are around the most. During these times, it is possible to be brought into the dramas of other people. In the book *The Celestine Prophecy*, the author makes his point concerning the new consciousness that has been entering the human world.

He introduces the nine insights of life, and the fourth insight deals with the control dramas that people use to control others. Sometimes we are pulled into these dramas very innocently and then other times we are brought into them for sheer control. This type of behavior will tend to bring on ill will, or even deep grudges in people's lives. The secret here is to realize when we are being brought into a control drama and then how to withdraw from it. Many times, these dramas are within family units and are very hard to avoid.

On the other hand, if they are within the school, social group, or athletic team they will not be as hard to withdraw from or correct the problem. In our modern day, we now have social media, i.e. Twitter, Facebook, to name two, and they can create many control situations in people's lives they do not even know personally. So, it is imperative that we be very careful in our participation in these forms of communication and not be pulled into these control dramas.

As always, I have consulted Dr. Weil on this subject, and while he doesn't approach it directly and head-on, he does talk about stress in our lives and what the result can be. The incidences that cause grudges also cause stress and that needs to be addressed.

The reason stress is so alarming in our lives is because it is very harmful to the brain and other organs. Now I am going to stick my neck out here and add some of my own thoughts to the stress subject: I believe that there is good stress and bad stress. Please understand that there is no complete elimination of stress in anyone's life. To eliminate stress, that means you are dead and buried.

With those thoughts, let me introduce "good stress" and "bad stress." "Good stress" is just simply that feeling of excitement and sense of urgency that enhances you with the thoughts and energy to accomplish any given task or goal. "Bad stress" results when the stress event goes from good to bad for any number of reasons. It could simply be a mechanical equipment difficulty or a control drama of a fellow worker. Regardless, the "good" boy will get you to victory while the "bad" boy can create failure.

I know everyone has seen the statement, "Your bad planning or procrastination is no excuse for me to get in a hurry, so chill!" In other words, do not create bad stress in my life because you have not planned well; that is not my concern. To prevent bad stress (1) Do complete prior planning on whatever is to be accomplished, (2) Have a detailed plan, (3.) Implement the plan with enough people to accomplish it, (4) Strive to meet the planned deadline, (5) Finish on time and recognize the team's efforts. Wow, that sounds like a good-stress project to me.

In referring to another strong source concerning this subject, I really like what Napoleon Hill says when he talks about the ownership of our thoughts. He says, "You have absolute control over but one thing, and that is your thoughts. This is the most significant and inspiring of all facts known to man! It reflects man's divine nature. This divine prerogative is the sole means by which you may control your own destiny. If you fail to control your own mind, you may be sure you will control nothing else. If you must be careless with your possessions, let it be in connection with material things. *Your mind is your spiritual estate!* Protect and use it with the care to which divine royalty is entitled. You were given a willpower for this purpose."

Please make every effort to eliminate grudges in your life. If you do, I promise that life will be better and, I know, healthier, both physically and mentally.

"Some Refreshing News from the Sport of Triathlon, for a Change!" 9.30.2005

Well despite the sport and all the stupid politics that goes on, there are some very good things going on. Recently I received a copy of the *Home Life Magazine*, actually the same day I received a copy of the totally bad rag, *Triathlon Times* sent by USA Triathlon. The magazines are in such contrast and it seemed ironic that they would come on the same day.

It was like getting a special message from George Carlin and Bill Graham all on the same day. Tri Times is such a waste of those beautiful trees that grow somewhere and are ruthlessly cut down to accommodate useless information published by Tri Times. On the other hand, there is hope on this green earth with such feel-good publications as the Home Life.

So, with that being said I would like to convey some of the great points that were brought out in this article about one of the most outstanding female triathletes the sport has been blessed with. The article really struck close to home for me since I have had some close-up dealings with some of the "elite" athletes of the sport.

While most of the experiences have been very good, the bad has been worse than bad. I will not dwell on the bad this morning since I am feeling good and will dwell on the bad some morning when I really feel like ragging some of the scum in the sport.

The good news about Barb and her husband, Loren, is that they appear to have their priorities in good order and represent the best in our society. It is so refreshing to see this generation set their goals and stick to their guns, no matter the consequences. Barb states, "My relationship with God is definitely number one in my life, and number two is my relationship with [my husband] Loren, the triathlon can take a back seat." "People will say that you're never going to be as good a triathlete if you don't put it as your number one priority, and you have to sacrifice everything for it." Barb adds, "But I think if you're not right with God first, then nothing else is going to be right in your life."

Barb has enjoyed the great outdoors her whole life. She grew up in Casper, Wyoming, starting her swimming, biking and running when she was eight years old. Her mother enrolled her in swimming very early and has been a strong influence on her athletic life. Her mother even started doing triathlons at the ripe ol' age of fifty-four herself and is still competing at sixty-one. The story goes on to say that Barb met her future husband through a cycling club in Jackson, Wyoming. A match made in heaven, with both understanding the great outdoors and what it took to compete on the international level. They married eight months later and have become a great triathlon team, with Barb competing, and Loren being her strong support in coaching, managing, and the technical aspects needed to compete in three disciplines. They have learned to counter act each other's weaknesses with their strengths, and it has paid off handsomely for them, both on and off the field of competition. While Barb has a long list of accomplishments, to include being on the Olympic team in 2004, she always goes back to the strong feeling of being right with God and keeping her priorities in life straight.

For the future, Barb has decided to retire from racing triathlon and will move forward in life, to the next step. They will focus their time now on building their family. They will continue in the sport of triathlon with camps, clinics and spreading the word of how to keep your priorities straight and still be one of the best in the world.

We wish them well and thank them for all they have done for our sport.

"Hero? Not!" 5.7.2013

Sometimes things come up that bug me, not to be confused with anger or disgust, they just "bug" me. Bugging is not a completely defined word and must be a slang word for pissed off, angry, befuddled, confused, or just wonder why about something not to be confused with curiosity. So, with that said I must say I am "bugged" about the recent announcement that professional basketball player Jason Collins came roaring out of the closet with the proclamation that he is gay. With all the comments by so called prominent people they are declaring him a "hero" and that really bugs me.

Okay now let me explain that I don't care whether someone is or isn't gay, that is their business, but why do I have to see news items revolved around this personal proclamation? While he is the first professional athlete to come out (meaning that other sports must also have gay men or women) of the closet he comes from a professional sport that I care nothing about, so I have no axe to grind here.

Coach Bobby Knight once said it best when he said he had rather watch two frogs making love than a professional basketball game, and I must confess that is also my feeling. My point of the day is this is not a heroic act, it is just a confession of a very personal thing and I hope the press has got their fill of it. Of course, now I expect a nice thick hard bound book to come out giving all the dirty details. Stay tuned!

While I am at it, a couple of articles in the sports pages carried some quotes from Dallas Cowboy owner Jerry Jones. Tony Romo stated to the loyal Cowboy fans that rather than be just a statistical leader amongst the previous Cowboy quarterbacks, he was going to work harder to become a "win" the critical games type quarterback. To do this he is going to adapt Payton Manning type work ethics. This means for his new contract of $105 million he is going to work out in the off season and spend more hours practicing so he will become the winner the fans expect.

You see Romo is a great quarterback, just like Hall of Famer Fran Tarkenton was but they have two things in common: they have never won a Super Bowl. This is the point of measurement that is used in all pro football quarterbacks. While Tarkenton took the Vikings to three Super Bowls he never won one. In the case of Romo he has never made it to the big show and has the distinction of losing the big games. Now what bugs me about this is that Romo is being paid this big money and Mr. Jones is so proud that he is going to work over time in the coming years. But as I write this it will be safe to say that no matter the amount of time he puts in on the field he will never win the big one! Now Mr. Tony man prove me wrong! As a life-long Cowboy fan who has turned North to watch a real championship quarterback in Peyton Manning, it would be fun to see Romo win in the Jerry Bowl!

God save the King!

Notes:

CHAPTER 9

Passion in Life

Live life to the fullest and focus on the positive.

—Matt Cameron

Passion in Life: While I know many readers at first glance may confuse this point of my life with that of point five, and even though one would probably have a passion within the normal sex drive, that is not what I am referring to in this point.

This point is one that I have recognized within my life for some time. I have found there are natural passions for some things in life, and then there are acquired passions. Neither one is more right than the other, but they do exist. Two good examples in my life have to do with natural and acquired, so I use them to illustrate my point.

When I was two years old, I recall running for the sake of just running, and then as I got older, exercise became a natural passion of mine. As I have aged in life that passion has never stopped, so no matter the form of sport or exercise I always have passion for it. Examples of this are in football, track, handball, bowling, endurance running, swimming, biking, and running in a triathlon.

Then on the opposite side of the scale of passion, my profession revealed passions that I feel were learned and experienced and not natural. Since I did not have the real desire to be a doctor, lawyer, engineer, chef, or anything specific, I realized I must find something that I really liked to do and then, much to my surprise, the passion came along. Even though my college training and degree was in business administration and marketing, I really was not sure that was the area I wanted to spend my life in.

So, I tried something else after leaving active duty that seemed to wake me up on where I needed to be. Of course, I had the desire to work and earn a living for my young, growing family but I can honestly say I did not have a passion for any particular thing.

After experimenting within one phase of the business world, I discovered that sales or marketing appealed to me very much, and after doing some research, I found the income potential was very good in the sales or marketing field. My first sales job seemed to awaken the ability to sell products, and therefore, providing me with a great income. As I progressed into the industrial packaging and material handling industries, I found my methods of selling were very effective, and they exemplified my passion for selling. Then my entrepreneurial spirits came alive, and I wanted to create my own business. This led to a grand total of $150 million in sales and ten small businesses that I founded over the years.

On the natural side of passion, I feel my athletic ventures have exemplified my natural passion activities in my life. When I was very young, I discovered I like to run a lot. As I mentioned above, my mother used to tell me that when I was two years old, I would run through the park seemingly forever.

She said it was not like I was trying to run away from her or anything, but I just liked to run.

As I went back into my memory banks, I did remember running in a park up in the Texas Panhandle at a town called Pampa, Texas. My mother told me I was two at the time when we lived there. I would guess that is one of my earliest memories, and it had to do with exercise.

When I was seven, I remember competing in a run-through game at school where you run through a bunch of people, and the last one standing was the victor. I always won those contests, since I was the fastest in the class and the others could not tackle me. This passion for exercise followed me all the way up to organized athletics such as football and track. These sports were so good to me that they provided me with full scholarships to college.

Many times as I watch athletes leave organized athletics and have no infrastructure or coaches to push them on, they quit all forms of athletics (could this possibly be they have no natural passion but have a learned passion for athletics?) and let their health go. As I left the college athletic setting, I wanted to keep my body in shape, but I still wanted to compete in something.

After being introduced to handball while on military duty, I followed through with it after leaving active duty and played in competitive matches, both tournament and training for twelve years. My next passion was to try some endurance running while entering short road races and later marathons. Then to do more cross-training for my body, I transitioned to triathlon. My endurance athletics in these two sports has been going on for thirty-eight years, and I feel will remain with me for many more.

Also, to be considered in the passion point is the possibility one could have a natural and acquired passion in life. In my case, I had enrolled in the ROTC program when I entered college, knowing I would wear a military uniform some of the time, and then when I got my degree, I would be required to go on active duty for no less than two years. My justification for this decision was not based on passion but simply on the fact I would be an officer in the US Army and would gain valuable experience for my civilian occupation.

After two years in ROTC, before you advance to the next and concluding two years, you must sign a contract, plus you must pass the physical. Of course, here I was a very active scholarship football player and track runner, so passing the physical exam was a simple walk through. Ooops, wrong! Because of a serious middle ear infection when I was a teenager, I had lost considerable hearing in my left ear. Due to this hearing loss, I was given a profile three on hearing. The requirement was a one across the board on all health ratings established by the US Army.

While I had an acquired passion to serve in the military, I now had a true passion to pass the physical exam, get my degree and commission, and then serve on active duty in a combat arm. So, I made every effort to do this, and even with a profile three, I was allowed to enter the third and fourth year of ROTC.

After receiving my bachelor's degree, I was commissioned a second lieutenant in the active US Army. I was able to serve in two command positions on active duty, with one hundred-sixty men and four officers under my command.

While my intentions were never to stay on active duty for more than three years, I did decide to remain in the Active

Reserves, and along the way, I served in two more commands and retired after twenty-four and a half years as a lieutenant colonel. My military service gave me an opportunity to serve my country, have awesome leadership training, and gain tremendous experience in leadership principles. I also saw and felt a tremendous passion to serve in the US Army, which had to be an acquired passion.

While I do believe that life passes through many phases of passion, I feel that in looking at healthy ageless living, one must maintain some form of passion for life in general. As I have aged, I have noticed the people around me in my age group seem to have lost the edge of passion. When I find articles about the passion within a ninety-year-old who wants to jump out of an airplane, I get excited. Turns out number forty-one President George H.W. Bush did this when he turned ninety and it was always a passion of his.

The challenge I present to my readers through this book is that there is an acknowledgement of passion within your life and that you take the time to find it and use it for a better life. It is there for us, so go get it!

"Aging Perception" 9.29.2012

Not a day goes by that I don't get into some kind of conversation about age and aging. Fact is it is mostly about my age and aging! For some reason I am the target of those who have a perception of what someone should look, or act like at a certain age. The remarks are, "you sure do not look your age" or "aging has been nice to you" or "how does it feel to be seventy-three?" or "I bet you whip up on your fellow age groupers when you race!"

My response is simple and honest with a thanks for the kind words and I am flattered. In response to the question how it feels the answer is great! But I do remind them if they look around, they will see very few things that are seventy-three and every one of my moving parts are that old.

The appliances in the house are not that old, your auto and its components are not that old, most of your friends are not that old, and even most of the trees are not that old. So, I guess that covers it all except for whipping up on my fellow age groupers. Fact of the matter is I do not whip up on them, and the ones that I raced against when we were younger that beat me then, are still beating me now, if they are still seriously racing.

Now what has motivated me to write about this sordid subject, that just never seems to go away, is an article I read the other day about Tom Osborne, the retiring athletic director at the University of Nebraska. While he spent his younger days as one of the most successful major college coaches at Nebraska he came back as the athletic director at the age of seventy. The program had gone south due to bad leadership, etc., so he was asked to come in and work his magic.

This he did and brought the Huskers back to their winning ways during his watch. Now what really drew my attention to the article was what he said as the reason for retiring from this position at seventy-five. He says, and I quote,

At some point, whether you're able to function or not, just the perception that you're getting old can get in the way. I don't want to be one of those guys everybody is walking around wringing their hands trying to figure out what are we going to do with him?

Funny thing is he has no health issues and considers himself healthier than when he was elected to Congress after his coaching days. So, here we go again, out to pasture with plenty of energy to graze. While I have experienced similar feelings and treatment, I blame it all on our youth obsessed society and real lack of respect for the seniors of our country. When I googled what world countries respected their elders the United States came in last, with Asian and Native American cultures were first.

Well here is the deal with me, as long as I can function, I am going head on strong into the world. While I know what I can do and can't do I will maximize all my efforts to what I can do. When I go into that giant triathlon event in the sky, I hope everyone says, "man that guy was so busy when he left, he must be resting now, and I wonder how many projects were left on his desk?" Go figure!!

"Psychic Income" 7.11.2010

Over the past twenty-one years it has been my pleasure, most of the time, to be in the business of race directing triathlons. This experience has been both rewarding and challenging, to say the least. The highs are way into the clouds while the lows are below the surface of the West Texas sandstone.

As I sit back and reflect on the twenty-first year of the Buffalo Springs Ironman 70.3, I still wonder what the attraction is to do this and why when it feels good, it feels good. So good in fact it is almost like sex or riding the hog, two of the most enjoyable things I can think of. When you spend the time preparing for the event starting one year out, then the last week before the event comes up and the unexpected happens. Now this is stuff you can't plan for, so you must shoot from the hip to get it done. Such things as weather, illness or injury to key volunteers, problems with the venue, unhappy athletes for one reason or the other, faulty equipment, etc.

You dig down deep and make it happen. You actually make it happen so well the athletes never know there was a problem of any kind. I have always said that the key to putting on a successful event is to have things happen behind the scenes that could put a negative on the event, but proper correction is done so smoothly that the athletes are not aware of it. My goal has always been to put on a race that all the athlete has to worry about is racing. If he or she has to worry about anything going on with the venue, then I have not done my job properly. Then the proof in the pudding is when the event comes to the last racer crossing the finish line and the remark, "great race!!" comes out of their mouth.

That is what I call psychic income and I am convinced, after talking to many race directors, that is what keeps all of us in the race directing business. When the racers come up to you and tell you what a great race you have just directed there is no better feeling.

Then the e-mails start coming in about how great the race is, etc. Even when you get the one sore head who thought the downhill on Spiral Staircase was too dangerous, you still sit back and say, "I love this sport and aren't downhills part of riding a bicycle?"

It was even suggested at one time that maybe we should take that downhill out of the race course, and my reply was simply, "over my dead body." I have ridden this downhill for over twenty years and have never come close to going down and I tell the racers to be careful and respectful of it or it might get the best of you. If they don't listen then they may go down, so when you are in my pre-race meeting please listen and ride the course with a good attitude and common sense.

On the same token I will have people tell me they love the challenge of the hills, especially Spiral Staircase, and they look forward to doing the race each year. This again puts large tokens of psychic income in the cash drawer of the mind and prompts me to come back and do it again and again. Fact is, planning is going on for 2012 right now as we speak. Thanks to all my readers out there who might also be competitors in the annual Buffalo Springs Lake Ironman 70.3 and if you are not, please take a ride to Lubbock and compete next year.

Notes:

CHAPTER 10

Embrace Adversity

I am not afraid of storms for I am learning to sail my ship.

—Louisa May Alcott

Embrace Adversity: As I look around my office and especially on the book shelves, I see all types of books and authors that offer many different kinds of opinions on various subjects, such as the following: Coach Bob Knight, *The Power of Negative Thinking*; George Carlin, *Napalm and Silly Putty*; Norman Vincent Peale, *The Power of Positive Thinking*; *Healthy Aging*, Dr. Andrew Weil; *Geronimo*, Mike Leach, and *Spartan Up*, Joe DeSena. But nothing really fits the bill for referencing the art of embracing adversity like the Holy Bible does.

My primary reference on point ten and the influence it has had on my life comes mostly from the King James Version of the Holy Bible. As I have ventured through life, there is no question I have experienced adversity many times over. In the beginning, I am sure I did not embrace it as I mentioned in ten, but I would say I certainly learned from it. I recall my first real adversity in life came when I was eight years old, and I was very sick with a bad kidney infection. I do remember being in the hospital, but I don't remember any pain as just being very sick.

Since that would be over sixty years ago, I am sure the doctors were still doing a lot of practicing on their seriously ill patients. I do know I was in that category, since the local Catholic priest came by my room and read the last rites. Funny thing about that is, I was raised a Presbyterian Protestant and had never ventured into a Catholic church. *But* I will say he must have done either a good job or a bad job since I did survive.

Maybe this was my first venture into adversity, and the incident happened with the priest to give me a good story to tell later in life. Regardless of the reason for this happening, I have always felt that being challenged with adversity is all part of life and how we come out of it has a lot to do with our future success and failures.

When I mention the Holy Bible concerning adversity, there are many stories within both testaments of how God has presented mankind with adversity and then reveals the results of this adversity. I also mention embracing adversity and I would like to elaborate on that to make my point and emphasize how important this point has made in my life. For me, the most revealing and illustrative story on embracing adversity comes from the story of Job in the Old Testament. While I think many people would like to mention the story of Jesus here as the top embracing adversity-for-growth story, I would like to emphasize that each story comes from different times and different settings. Job comes from the Old Testament and exemplifies the people of that time and describes just raw tough testimony as to the truth of God. While I do not intend for this to coast into a religious discussion, I feel the story of Job will really take more meaning when my discussion is completed.

In the book of Job, it begins with some tidbits about Job being a true and honest man with many assets and family. While this is all true, the rest of the story is that Satan is making a deal with the Lord to prove to him that Job is not as strong and true as it appears, and if everything is taken away from him, he will falter and deny God. Then when God agrees to allow Satan to do his harm on Job, he begins to lose everything. While Job did do some questioning on "Why me, Lord," he did not falter in his beliefs and stood strongly about his beliefs in God. Then the end of the story that many people forget is that because of Job's retaining the faith, all his losses were restored to him, including his livestock and family.

In reality, he had embraced the adversity to the extent that he'd asked for more, got it, then endured to the end of having everything restored back to him. Satan lost, Job won, and God was pleased!

In my life, I have experienced my own Job story, and because of that, I have had a strong testimony of God, and the challenge of adversity. My story had to do with my business and a person of the family that was involved in my business. It was a very disturbing time of my life and during the worst part of it, I got so stressed with the situation that I dropped to my knees and prayed to God that I was being tried very hard and the times were bad, but I wanted more adversity. I wanted to see what real strength I had, so I asked for more. Well, lo and behold, God answered my prayers and when I got to my business that day it got much worse. So, from this, three things happened: I knew that God answered prayers, and I knew that

I got stronger with embracing the adversity, and it became a great teaching and learning part of my life.

"Frequently Ask Questions (FAQ) After the Crash" 6.5.2011

The other day I got a note from a friend of mine asking how I was doing after the crash. My reply: Honestly it only hurts when I eat, sleep, stand, sit, slump, bathroom tricks, motorcycle tricks, bicycle tricks, sex (none at this time, so hurts more), see my blue balls in the mirror, shower, soak, drive, drink, swallow, itch, scratch, laugh, frown, barf, sneeze, spit, blow nose, clear throat, type, giggle, not get pissed off, get pissed off, see my friends, or even see my enemies. This is a great lesson in pain tolerance without pain pills, so I am really growing out of this adventure. The good news is that my friend was understanding, and I feel better every day. My full recovery is getting closer!!

"Pity Party, Not" 6.5.2011

If you ride a bicycle long enough two things will happen, you crash for sure and then some time later you crash again. My eighth crash over a twenty-eight-year period was a little over a week ago and it turned out to be my worst. Aside from a slightly fractured pelvis, heavily bruised hip, huge bump on top of my head (with helmet), road rash, broken rib, stitches in cut on arm, bruising from hip to bottom of my left foot, everything is fine.

After a night in the hospital I was assured that I would be good as new in eight weeks. Little did they know I have plans for six weeks so my body is working on it now. The following blogs will cover my experiences with this event, and how it fits into the idea of transitioning life to accommodate current events. This is not going to be a pity party but the realizations of the challenges that face us in life and what we can go about them. Let's have some fun with this...I already have!

"Plan B" 5.27.2013

When I look at my library, I notice all forms of books from many different authors. It is almost as if I am schizophrenic or something, as they range from George Carlin to the King James Version of the Holy Bible. But two of the authors really stand out and probably reveal something about my deep inner thoughts, namely Norman Vincent Peale with *The Power of Positive Thinking* and Bobby Knight, *The Power of Negative Thinking* both stand tall on my shelves.

Does that make me positive or negative or do I see the point of each? Good question but I would say my attempt to do my eighth Ironman triathlon last weekend was a combination of positive/negative and the results was a total mess. I had not waited ten years to do my next Ironman to have it end the way it did. I had worked extremely hard, probably the hardest ever, to do well in this event and even had some kind of weird thoughts I might possibly make it to Kona. How wrong I was on that and the realization of what had happened this day came to my thick head sometime in the next few days after the event.

What I could say is at the start it was just too rough and overpowering with 2,200 athletes kicking, clawing, biting, punching, kicking, cussing, and swimming like fish, around me. Even though this was true it was not the reason for my dismal swimming performance. The fact is my swimming sucks and has sucked all my thirty years of doing triathlons. However, on this day the realization set in that I had gotten away with it over the years with simple out right athleticism and it had overpowered my inadequate swim position and stroke with my football mentality of getting through it with my physical athletic ability no matter what it looked like. BAM, BAM go for it!!

BUT!! Alas on this day I presented the triathlon world with a completely new look, I was now seventy-four years old and had never done this distance at this age. What I found was that my mind was still athletic, but my body was not and low and behold my arms just gave out. No matter how much I thought mind over matter, and I am strong, and get out of my way swimmers I am still in it, it just wasn't reality. So, when I was invited by the authorities to leave the water I did so with relief and joy, by God I had not drowned and could still walk (but not on water!!).

So, I have re-examined my future in triathlon and have promised myself I will only enter open water swim events that allow wetsuits and will do mostly sprint pool swim events.

I can still stay in very good shape and have more time for other things. While the Ironman distance is still the ultimate, I have my eight and the tat on the left arm, so why do I need any more?

This coming weekend I will be doing my three-hundred-fiftieth triathlon at the infamous Milkman Triathlon and the swim is five-hundred yards with a wetsuit, so beware I am going to enjoy this fun!

Notes:

CHAPTER 11

Family and Friends

The love of family and the admiration of friends is much more important than wealth and privilege.

—Charles Kurait

Family and Friends: While this point may be the last, it is sure not the least because of its position. As I mentioned earlier, I was sitting in a café when I wrote the first list out on a paper napkin. As I went along for a few years, I added the last ones, and when I draw my circle of the eleven points, each one will have to be on the circle in equal sizes or equal proportions. They are all important and have been part of my life.

I am sure more would argue that family is more important than friends so there must be an emphasis on that. While I would not argue this point, I believe they both have equal importance in my mind. I do agree they have a different kind of importance.

Sometimes, it is hard to be friends with blood relatives, while it is also hard to put friends in the same amount of priority as family. So, with those points put forth on number eleven, I would like to say families are most important to healthy ageless living. They can be such an influence that sometimes sad or hurtful things happen within a family.

I believe no matter how much effort we put forth toward our immediate families, we can probably never do more than needs to be done. When my immediate family—sister, mother, and father—all passed away way too early in our lives, I know it left a lot that needed to be said before they passed. So, based on that, my advice to anyone with family still living, it would be good to restore any estrangement that exists. If that is not entirely possible for whatever reason, then a resolution in your mind should make the time easier.

I do know that there are many days that go by I would like to talk with my mother and my dad, just to cover some things that were never addressed. But the good side is I have many good memories of both my parents, and it is great to retrieve them in my mind. I try to always go for the positive side from my childhood up to my adulthood and use the positives for a better life.

While friendships are very important, it is very disturbing when they are lost. Please recall earlier about my doctor saying I was going to be a very lonely man because I was going to outlive all my friends. Well, I have outlived over a dozen of my friends so far, and two of these were my best friends. I must say the doctor was right. I am learning the hard way you don't just go out and make new best friends with ease, so when you lose one for whatever reason, it makes it very lonely. Do not take for granted your friendships since they are very important to your healthy ageless living.

In conclusion, I would like to share a request given by Dr. Weil concerning legacy and the act of writing an ethical will. An ordinary will normally concerns the disposition of one's material possessions at the time of death. An ethical will has to do with non-material gifts: the values and life lessons you wish to leave to others.

In *Healthy Aging*, Dr. Weil has included his ethical will, and just reading it makes it worthwhile to buy this book. Please note the next to last paragraph of his ethical will, and you will see the value. He says: "Finally, I want to extend to you my blessings and wishes for graceful, healthy aging as you advance in years. I hope you will discover and enjoy the benefits aging can bring: wisdom, depth of character, the smoothing out of what is rough and harsh, the evaporation of what is inconsequential, and the concentration of true worth." The good news here is that you do not need to be an attorney to write this will since it comes straight from the heart, and there is nothing to fight over amongst the heirs.

Please understand the one for sure conclusion is when you age, you do not have to grow old, but it is more fun when you do, since that means you are still above ground!

"Losing Something" 1.19.2015

When I lose my glasses or cell phone that is a loss that makes me instantly mad or upset, to say the least. Then when I lose something of more value or importance to me, that causes a sinking, empty feeling that lingers on for some time. It has been two weeks since Mr. Buffman, our fourteen-year-old Boston Terrier died in his sleep, and I am finding I still miss him a lot. When he played with the other dogs the little shorty Bob use to bite Buffman's back legs to aggravate him. He would be patient at first then would finally take charge and let Bob have it with a few snips and a deep growl.

Now I am noticing that Squeaky, Marley and Bob are really missing him and for at least a week they only ate half of what they usually eat. While I am not putting as much food out for them, they are at least eating like normal now. The other thing I have noticed is far less poop in the back yard since the poop pickup patrol comes on my watch. I have always thought when one of these four died the easy thing to do would be to go out and buy another one, but now I know while I can do that it would not really replace the Buffman. It would just be another dog with its own personality and attitude.

Possibly the same is true of lost loves or friendships, you just don't go running out finding the same thing you have experienced overnight and the same is true of losing long time close friends or relatives. I have lost a couple of my best friends over the past few years and it was very hard to realize, on the other hand I have lost some friends from my early years and the loss does not seem that drastic. Within the last two weeks I have lost two of my old friends from my church and hand ball days, and since I had not seen them recently the loss didn't seem as drastic, so as the world turns!! Now to get out there and see all my old friends hopefully not to say goodbye but to say, hello how are you today!!

"Webster Says!" 5.24.2008

When you are at a loss for words there is always one great resource to go to for guidance, the Webster's Dictionary. You know the old saying, "well Webster says, etc." In consulting Webster, I find the following definition for the word friend.

Friend(s), a person to whom one is attached by affection: an intimate acquaintance; one well inclined toward a cause, as a friend of democracy. Friendship(s), intimacy and mutual attachment; a friendly relationship, especially one of long standing.'

Well this past weekend we were afforded the opportunity to enjoy some of our friends from the Show Me State, Missouri. Mark & Amy Livesay, Clint & Shandra Chapman ventured to Lubbock to compete in the Buffman and Squeaky Triathlon.

All four of these folks competed and enjoyed the challenges and misery of the swim, bike and run event held at Buffalo Springs Lake. Not only did they travel (almost nine-hundred- miles) to Lubbock but they stayed with us in Ransom Canyon.

Over the years we have had many athletes and friends stay with us during events, and we enjoy them all, but this group (any number over two is a group) brought some special aura to the canyons and our household. While Amy and Mark both won their age groups, Shandra and Clint showed the canyons that they could survive the wrath of dry heat and challenging hills, both with strong finishes.

Since these folks put on a series of very high-quality races, the UltraMax races in Missouri, we had to really do our stuff to show them a great triathlon race venue. We feel that the venue, the volunteers, the sponsors, and everyone connected with the event made this happen. They were very complimentary of the entire production and promised to come back for the big one in June 2007 (I thought this blog was written in 2008?). We welcome them with open arms.

The other point I would like to make about these friends is that they are about the age of my own children and regardless of our age difference we had a great time together and age meant nothing. But the other big point I would like to make is that every parent would like for their children to be good people and offer positive vibes to the world.

Well I can assure the parents of these four young adults, they can be really proud of their children. My hope would be that my four children offer the same high quality of attitude and hope to the world (and I believe they do) that these four do. They display all the attributes a parent would want in their children: integrity, honesty, dedication, responsible, physically fit, intellectually fit, sense of humor, progressive attitude towards growth, always accepting the challenge to move out of their comfort zones for success, plus they even clean up after themselves, and on and on! Congrats to them and we look forward to seeing them again.

Notes:

Bibliography

Campbell, Joseph. *The Power of Myth*. New York: Doubleday, 1988.

Hill, Napoleon. *Think and Grow Rich*. USA: Ballantine Publishing, 1960.

Hubbard, L. Rob. *Dianetics*. Los Angeles: Bridge Publications, 1985.

Leach, Mike. *Geronimo* New York: Gallery Books, division of Simon & Schuster, 2014.

Redfield, James. *The Celestine Prophecy*. USA: Time Warner Co., 1993.

Sheehan, George. *Running and Being*. New York: Simon & Schuster, 1978.

Torian, Ashly, and Jim Waldsmith. Join Me in the E.N.D. Zone.

Weil, Andrew, M.D. *Healthy Aging*. New York: Random House Inc., 2005.

Connect with Me

Please visit my website at
http://fasttwitchmind.blogspot.com/.

You can find me on Facebook at
https://www.facebook.com/mike.greer.5030.

I'd love a follow on my Amazon page as well at:
https://amzn.to/2ueC7dO.